JULIA CARROLL

B.F.A., M.A., A.T.C.

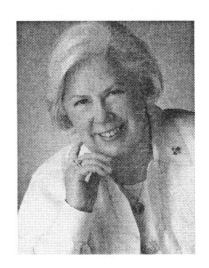

HEALING H'ARTS

SPIRITUAL SHAMAN SECRETS

For information on workshops or for personal counseling please write or email the following:

Julia Carroll, M.A., A.T.C.
P.O. Box 270957
Houston, Texas 77277-0957
E-mail: jcarroll@wt.net

Book design by Gail's Graphics

PUBLISHED BY
Reiki Touch Institute of Holistic Medicine™ Publishing
P.O. Box 270957
Houston, Texas 77277-0957
E-mail: jcarroll@wt.net

ISBN: 0-615-12913-7

Library of Congress Control Number: 2005927175

Printed in the United States of America

Healing H'Arts
Spiritual Shaman Secrets
Fifty Years of Personal Experiences Woven with Patterns of Healing

Acupressure

Appearances

Art Therapy

Auras

Balancing Chakras

Cancer

Crystals

Death and Dying

Etheric Surgery

Exorcisms

Hearts

Huna and Kahunas

Meditation

Money

Native American Lore

Protections

Psychometry

Psychology

Psychic Surgery

Regression

Reiki Touch™ Therapy

Shamanism

Stress Management

Truth

Visual Imagery

Other books by Julia Carroll

REIKI TOUCH
by Judy-Carol Stewart (aka Julia Carroll)

Soon to be published

HEALED BY LIGHT – 2005
REIKI TOUCH (3rd Edition) – 2006
LAKSHMI – 2006

"Muchos son los estudiosos que se han dedicado a examinar dicho fenomeno, y entre ellos surge la maestra Julia Carroll experta en metodos revitalizadores de la salud."
— El Universal - El Gran Diario De Mexico - Mexico, D.F. - Agosto de 1993

"Julia Carroll has a deep desire to be of help to her fellow human beings and is vitally interested in the healing of the whole person. Julia has made a deep study of methods of healing and from a personal touch we discovered she has a healing touch."
— J. Sig and Janie Paulson, (late) Houston, Texas Unity of Christianity Ministers

"The method of Reiki Touch™ Therapy uses ageless principles and power, and concerns itself with alignment of the body, mind and spirit. The focus here is on wellness, which is the absence of disease, rather than on a reversal of pathological changes; such reversals are irrelevant in a state of wellness. Herein lies the distinction between healing and curing. This is a tool of profound significance and endless potential."
— M. Truett Bridges, Jr., M.D., Acupuncturist, Reiki Master

"Results: Comparing before and after measures of the quantitative data, anxiety was significantly reduced (t_{22} = 2.45, P = .02). Systolic blood pressure dropped significantly ($F_{2,44}$ = 6.60, P = .003). Salivary IgA levels rose significantly (t_{19} = 2.33, P = .03)."
— Alternative Therapies in Health and Medicine, A Peer-Reviewed Journal, March/April 2002, Volume 8, No. 2 (Reiki Touch Therapy Research)

"The findings of a single Reiki session has an effect on decreasing perceived anxiety, increasing signs of relaxation, and increasing humoral immunological functioning through an increase of IgA. There were changes in the individual's biochemical and psychological responses."
— Blackwell Science Ltd., UK 2001 (Reiki Touch Therapy Research)

"Reiki Touch Therapy is the forefront of combining traditional and holistic medicine for the modern individual."
— Emerging Lifestyles Magazine, Vol. 4, No. 12, September 2002

CONTENTS

Section Three: **SPIRIT**

Foreword

Carol E. Parrish-Harra, PhD

ealing H'Arts is an exciting book about impressive events in both spiritual and physical realities. Julia Carroll relates experiences in and out of body with a grace that determines the depth of her reality. Yet, through it all, you are intrigued by her story.

Living in a world that needs healing, seeks healing and prays for healing, when it comes, we rejoice and give thanks. When it does not happen, we struggle to understand why. What else could we have done? As more and more of us take healing workshops, passionately wanting to be a part of the healing reality rather than to be found standing by unable to help, we stretch into new dimensions.

This is such a story: one that spans fifty years and stretches around the planet. We travel with Julia as she is challenged and as she challenges the forces that may or may not bring change to the physical or emotional nature of one in need. The world of today is experiencing many phases of belief, doubt, quest and experimentation—all at the same time. We cannot be classified simply by any one term. We are both the experimenters and the seekers trying a variety of approaches to find our way to well being.

In a world of such rapidly expanding ideas, we hunt for the unique blend of black and white, truth and untruth, myth and mystery that we can accept and own. We each frame our reality with our personal experiences when we judge the stories of others from that perspective. Knowing this, I suggest that as you read *Healing H'Arts*, prepare to adjust your rational mind, for here you will venture into realities practiced by those individuals who experience them.

As Julia colorfully describes her journeys into other realities, the list of extraordinary healings fills our hearts. Others, perhaps just as remarkable, touch us when healing does not happen on the physical but carries us along to explore an awareness of after-life states. Protected stories of after-life reveal mysteries that lie in this hidden space. The greatest healing may be that which releases the soul from bondage. Julia shines a ray of light into that understanding.

Not everyone can journey here. Yet for those who seek hope and healing and would persist in the long stretch that is required of aspiring disciples, rich wonder is the reward. For those who serve tirelessly while persisting to hope that the world will catch up, this volume can provide assurance and strengthen the dedicated to carry on.

Fortunately we live in a renaissance period that is stimulating the collective consciousness to explore an ever-expanding field of information. The emergence of new techniques and the renewal of old are hard to dismiss. The reappearance of laying-on-of-hands, as well as Reiki Touch™—a similar Japanese approach—and the effectiveness of prayer and invocations intrigues the inquiring mind.

If we can come to think in terms of parallel realities, with life occurring in each of a band of frequencies, it may help. As we are accustomed to dialing television channels 3, 7 or 9 and readily accepting a new program on each, some are learning to attune to different realities, finding happenings on each. In her sharing, Julia Carroll reveals she has traveled vast airwaves and experienced much. Now she opens her journal for us to see just how far her exploration has led her. Most healers share some part of such experiences, but not as extensively.

A lovely, well-educated woman, widely traveled and highly regarded, Julia willingly shares all that she does. Why does she tell us these stories of overlapping realities? Might it be that the adventurer wants us to know? Think of the astronauts as they return from outer space. Can they *not* speak of the wonders they have found?

So it is, I believe, with our author. Julia Carroll has spent fifty years caring and serving. This seeker has followed healing techniques around the world in order to observe, to learn, to experience and to practice. Guided to a number of profound individuals—known and unknown to the public—she has amassed new awareness, skills and accomplishments. A dedicated follower of her Guru, Julia is recognized as a credible healer by both the establishment and the fringe element, as she acknowledges. Due to her willingness to find what worked and use it whether others understood it or not, she has worked and waited. Now she tells her story and ah ha!—we have a window through which to view these unique events.

Both as a spiritual teacher and as a death-and-dying counselor, I realize the power of transformative moments. Most of these may seem more of a blessing for the patient, perhaps, than the healer. I have come to know, however, this is not the usual situation. I believe we come to appreciate such sacred moments are for both parties—for all who are present—and are never easy to share with others. It is not possible to re-create the charge, the dynamics, the pain and joy of such profound and powerful spiritual high-points. We can only ponder them. This book is like that. It is to be pondered and applauded.

And as you do so, allow your inner presence to expand, to delight and to glow with the stories of healings and happenings that have changed the individuals to whom they have occurred. No, we cannot all do these things, but we can all rejoice that they have been done.

When a revival of spiritual healing began in the seventies, many looked away in disdain. Now we have techniques taught to nurses and practitioners who have demonstrated their power and their benefits.

Reiki Touch™ and other natural modalities have proven to make a difference. Nurses, psychologists and some physicians have forged new paths in their quest for effective tools. On the cutting edge are those who think out of the box. Today we call these pioneers "holistic," while in times past they would simply have been called "holy."

This recording of events experienced by our author, while educated to society's norm, nevertheless demonstrates the significance of life-giving energy. She studied with those who actually did psychic surgery and etheric cleansing, whether or not they were board certified. Her love of the Divine surrounded her as it led her to indigenous methodologies embraced by few.

We are learning from and emboldened by those who dare to venture further and further from limitation to swim in the energy of the Great Life. Read on, and congratulate Julia Carroll that she has crossed the line into a healing energy that knows no bounds.

As one healer to another,
Carol

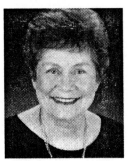

Carol E. Parrish-Harra, PhD, Mystic, Author, Teacher, Counselor, Minister, is the founder and spiritual director of the community of Sparrow Hawk Village, minister of Light of Christ Community Church and Dean of its seminary, Sancta Sophia.

Carol's latest book is *Adventure in Meditation - Spirituality for the 21st Century.* She has also authored *The New Dictionary of Spiritual Thought, The New Age Handbook on Death and Dying,* her autobiography; *Messengers of Hope* and others. Her most recent honor is the Earl Award for Religious Futurist of the Year for "exceptional achievement in the field of religious future activities."

Sparrow Hawk Village
11 Summit Ridge Drive
Tahlequah, Oklahoma 74464
www.sanctasophia.org

Introduction

Who knew? A curious nine-year-old, sitting in church, trying to be still (so she wouldn't be deprived of dessert later) and halfway listening to a visiting missionary. The missionary was a diminutive lady from China poignantly expressing her people's plight of physical and spiritual hunger.

I was struck in a place in my body, gripped and given my future in a brief, invisible moment in time. It was as if my future were passing before my young eyes. From that moment on I "knew" that I would be a healer and go around the world and heal people. Now, my nine-year-old Southern Baptist self truly thought that she would be a missionary, just like the little Chinese lady.

It did not happen quite that way. However, on that very Sunday after church, I announced to anyone who would listen that I was a healer, and I was going to go around the world and heal people when I grew up. The comments were supportive and inspiring; "go away little girl, go play with your dolls, I'm busy now," and other comments of that ilk.

I would listen to conversations and anytime I heard someone say that they were not feeling well, I would rush up to them and ask if I could pray for their health. My fervor was so great and if they were feeling really bad, then they would say yes. My little nine-year-old knees hit the floor beside my bed every night with sincere and believing prayers for that person's health.

The next day, if I happened to see them, I had to instantly know how they felt, because I was positive that the prayers worked. They would report that yes, they did feel better, but the doctor had given them a shot, or that the prescription from the doctor finally kicked in. These words would ring in my head for decades. No matter how dedicated, talented and skilled I became in my healing work, the traditional medical community was "God." I quickly perceived that I was to work "outside the box" and that my level of validation would be second, if that, to the MDs'. At least I learned early where I stood. Thank goodness it did not stop me.

The following pages reveal my journey from that nine-year-old child, through decades of holistic and metaphysical healing practices. Even though I did gather, along the way, a few letters after my name, it was to open doors to arenas into which I would have been denied .

Traditional medical communities now have a complementary or alternative office in every hospital. It has been mandated. Reason? Because the world population tired of all the surgeries, chemicals, scar tissue and side effects, and began to spend money on alternative and holistic practices, to the tune of $60 to $90 billion dollars per year. All of a sudden the pharmaceutical companies wanted to make the vitamins and supplements and state the dosage and use. Now they are and in some ways that is a good thing. It is, I think, an acceptance of the changes going on in the world.

This journey has taken me around the world several times into realms of which I never before dreamt. The exposure to cultures, creeds, belief systems and wellness programs are multitudinous. I am fortunate to have trained with the best healers of all kinds in the world. You will travel with me into the path of pain, sorrow, death and, with it all, great joy and amazement. I have been rewarded by it all and regret none of the experiences.

Understand clearly as you read these pages that the allopathic medical establishment, even with the current research to prove otherwise, considers these practices "fringe medicine." Allow me to increase an awareness of the posture of the psychopathology of fringe medicine.

Fringe medicine first has the premise that there is a desire to believe in the therapy and the therapist. It is often difficult to differentiate between a fringe therapy and a paranormal claim. Astrology, reflexology, psychic surgery and others put themselves into the category of alternative medicine, which incorporates osteopathy, acupuncture, homeopathy and others of like ilk. These all ask to be believed without the benefit or results of investigation or research.

Perhaps we should know that the traditional medical arena does want to know why people practice and use fringe medicine and does it work and when does it work. The word psychopathology is used in this discussion because some feel that a mental disorder or disease may be present in those who seek fringe medicine. Is it because of human psychology and physiological links between mind and body?

Dr. E. Freireich of the M.D. Anderson Cancer Center in Houston, Texas offers a "Freireich Experimental Plan." This plan enables virtually anyone to set himself up as a therapist who guarantees to produce beneficial results. He then produces a cartoon depicting a tongue in cheek analysis. However this plan explains a lot about how an impression of effectiveness can come about in fringe medicine.

Freireich continues with two requirements. One is a "treatment" of some sort. Second is that this treatment must be absolutely harmless. He states that conditions can be set up from almost any treatment to lead to a situation which can be determined as successful. Even if the disease or problem remains stable the treatment can be confirmed as successful.

Even if death occurs the fringe therapist can claim that the other medicines did not work and the fringe treatments were delayed too long, or applied too late.

What Dr. Freireich does state is that people often get better or worse for no particular reason. This is regardless of any treatment whatsoever, be it traditional or fringe medicine. He continues, saying that doctors and healers are not familiar enough with probability figures or the natural history of disease to make an informed judgement or to apply an assessment of therapeutic effectiveness. An example was an observation made by his young daughter, "Those trees surely are pushing the wind around."

Negative evidence has had little to no impact on fringe practitioners. One comment is: "Rogerian therapy has no set technique and no set procedures to follow." Another: "T'ai Chi teachers emphasize the impossibility of describing it in print." Yet another: "The Feldenkrais method is difficult to explain quickly and easily, with Feldenkrais himself saying that the first principle of his work is that there isn't any principle." Freireich sums up by suggesting that fringe medicine might work, and poses the question: "Does it matter?"

I have personally been involved with university-based studies and research which clinically document certain improvements and successes with various study subjects. Even then, we, myself as a holistic healer and the traditional medical practitioners, all agree that more research is needed in this field. Does it matter? You decide.

As you read the book just enjoy the journey. Know that these experiences are real, from real people with real situations. Travel with me from head to toe as patterns of healing are woven into people's bodies, minds and spirits.

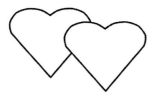

Gratitude

My gratitude is always first and foremost to my Guru, to Her Guru, to His Guru and the entire effulgent lineage of Siddha Masters in all their forms.

To my only child Mandy, and my grandchildren Bryn, Gabi and Will who give me the experiences of love, woven with attachment and detachment.

To my grandmother, Nannie, a traditional nurse and a folk healer who turned no one away; Pappy, my grandfather, who carried me on his shoulders so I could touch the stars; my parents, Gwyn and Sonny, who gave me karmic lessons from which to grow; to my brothers, Roy and Michael, who shielded and protected me as best they could, and my nieces and nephews who carry the healing patterns within and without.

To my aunts, uncles, cousins, with whom I shared sweet summers and still provide poignant memories.

To my dear friends, colleagues and mentors; a true family with sacred bonding.

To all my teachers, formal by name and informal by lessons.

And, to all, known and unknown, in body and out of familiar forms, who provided the experiences for this book.

I thank you again and again for providing the path of healing for me to serve God and mankind in this vast universe.

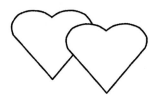

HEAD
Mother

I am an Aries and Aries rules the head, so perhaps I should not be so surprised that many head situations presented themselves to me. Frequently, in public lectures, people ask me if I have performed a miracle. Of course, I have not. But, God, through me, in Her Grace, has.

One miracle event was my mother. On a senior church trip my mother was walking across a street in New Orleans and tripped on a crack in the street. She fell face forward onto the nearby curb. Her movie star smile was altered as a couple of front teeth were knocked out. As the doctors were examining her, a shadowy image appeared on the x-rays. It was a brain tumor.

The next five years involved many surgeries and medical treatments. These years also involved much morphine, lots of nurses, and my dad taking care of her all day, every day. Her first surgery was about sixteen hours long. Her body temperature had to be lowered to below seventy degrees. Every time the surgeon would get to the part of the tumor in her brainstem, she would die on the operating table. So, they never, with that surgery or the ensuing ones, completely got the tumor.

Her left ear became completely deaf. She was in pain constantly or knocked out with drugs. Her life was basically over. Because of my family's negative view of holistic health, I was kept away. Completely. After about two and a half years a secret call informed me of my mother's location and of a surgery about to be performed. I made the trip and was greeted by a family member who sarcastically asked if I had come to "heal" Momma. The family did not want to let me in to see her; and even when I did manage to see her, I was not allowed to touch her.

She had been so drugged she did not recognize me. So I left. I did not return for a couple of years. My family was very clear that I was not wanted and that the work I did was "un-Christian" and more than likely just straight from the devil. My primary work was and is Reiki Touch™ Therapy. When I asked permission on an etheric level to enter my mother's space to send her healing, her Higher Self denied me. This perpetuated me staying away. It was her truth not to experience Reiki at that time.

I did travel to see her a few times over the years. Once, I drove into the driveway unannounced and walked into the house. My dad was there. The nurse had left. He was exhausted. Simply exhausted. My mother's mother was grieving and wringing her hands. Her primary duty was to sit beside my mother's bed, to pray and read the Bible to my mother. This lasted all day, every day. I stayed for three weeks, which allowed daddy to get some rest. I bathed my mother, changed her diapers and listened to her nonsensical conversation as the surgeries had left her speech in a jumbled mess. I sang to her and told her stories of my daughter and my travels. She responded as best she could.

Very soon after that visit she entered the hospital. One of those times when you "know" she will not leave. She was on several life support systems and the family had a meeting, without me, and decided that the life support systems should be removed. A date was set for that. It was around Christmas time. On Monday a nurse came in to wish mother "Merry Christmas" and to tell her she would be taking a couple of days off. Mother, in her defaulted speech, said, "Then I'll see you Wednesday." Just after that Mother commented to someone else, "Weren't the lights on the Christmas tree twinkly." Now, this is not a brain dead person. This is a person still having cognitive functioning. Yet, the doctor was going to allow the life support systems to be removed because there was "no hope of complete recovery." A side decision was made to just remove her feeding tube and starve her to death. She was just about gone anyway—so everyone said.

My grandmother fell to the floor, grabbed the doctor's knees and sobbed, "Please do not starve my baby to death." The doctor explained, in medical jargon, that this was best for my mother. Nannie and I both went into shock. Daddy and my brothers were very matter of fact that this was the way it was. After about six days of no food, no water and no medication she was still alive. It was time now, they said, to remove the life support systems.

I found an attorney who agreed with me that this was akin to murder and we obtained a court injunction and stopped the process. Later, the social worker at the hospital told me that they were secretly going to move Mother out because they did not want to be a party to this action. My dad was extremely angry. After all, the funeral was planned, the choir was ready, and the flowers were ordered. I also found out that somewhere in the not too distant shadows was "another woman." My dad said that he was having a hard time with Mother being ill. He was lonesome. It was a really hard time for him. I wonder how it was for her?

I went over to Mother's bed. She had atrophied a great deal, had no hair anywhere on her body, her face was very distorted from the illness, the treatments, Bell's Palsy, and the endurance of a five-year trauma. I leaned over and told her that I felt she knew what they were going to do to her and that I felt it was not her time to die. I needed her permission to do Reiki Touch Therapy on her. That it was the highest and the only thing I could do for her and that it would be a gift of healing, which could only have a positive result. She did not speak. But, she did open and shut her eyes several times, which I understood was a "yes."

That was on December 23. I pushed the hospital bed away from the wall and leaned my body against the wall and put my hands on my mother's head. I stayed there for about five hours. I did the same the next day. I had to return home to work, but came back the next weekend with other Reiki practitioners. We surrounded her for two days and did many, many hours of Reiki on her. By February there was no tumor, no cancer. The doctors said it was "delayed radiation" and "delayed chemotherapy."

Her speech returned, her memory returned; she said, "Didn't Mrs. Tompkins' son get married last October?" In October it was understood that mother was in a deep coma from which she'd never return. I got a physical therapist, a dentist, a hairdresser (her hair grew back), some new clothes and began a journey of wellness for my mother. At the end of February she had gone from a feeding tube to cutting up her own meat, opening her milk carton and feeding herself. She had gone from a catheter to a bedpan to getting up and walking to the bathroom by herself. She had gone from the range of motion physical therapy to walking down the hall to the physical therapy gym for her treatments.

By March she told Daddy, "Take me home." Too late, Daddy already had his next life planned and in place. He said that he could not. I brought her things, as many as possible, to the hospital room: her photos, reclining chair, TV. Now she was alone and very sad, watching *Wheel of Fortune* and *Jeopardy*. Her mother was there with her faithfully, every day. I was there every weekend, continuing the Reiki treatments. The family and the doctors were clearly perplexed. They did not know what to do about me or her. My very staunch Southern Baptist grand-mother was now sure that I had performed a miracle on her daughter. She thought it was a Buddhist thing and was really uncomfortable with that. I just explained to her that some things existed before Christ.

In mid-April, I had a telephone call requesting that I resume my work in New York. After about a week of preparing my mother that I was leaving for a couple of weeks, I went to New York. I left a tape recorder on auto reverse, playing *Amazing Grace*, on a very low volume for the entire time I was gone. On April 27, the nurse called and said that Mother had developed a cold, but she thought she would be fine, just wanted to let me know. I asked if I should return and the nurse said she thought it would be fine. I did not go. Things sometimes are the way things are.

On April 29 I awoke feeling a bit uneasy without being able to identify it. I was very particular as to what I wanted to wear. I took a long time and was very deliberate in my movements with makeup, hair and getting dressed. Even after I left my room I returned to recheck how I looked and considered chang-ing into something else. I finally was okay with how I was dressed and walked to another building in which a small celebration of April birthdays was being held. A celebrated and beloved Teacher of mine was the guest of honor. I smiled and joined the group. The uneasy thoughts left me.

As Happy Birthday songs were wafting through the air, a lady came and told me there was a phone call for me. I asked if I could return it later, as I was enjoying the celebratory tone of the moment. She looked into my eyes and sug-gested that I take this call. Something stirred inside, but no connection as to what it was. I took the receiver. It was Sharon, my secretary in Houston. She said that my mother had just passed away and that I should return home right away. I lightly laughed, and said that my mother was fine and asked the real rea-son for her call. Sharon said that Daddy had just called her and mother had left her body at 11 A.M, about twenty minutes prior to the call. Sharon offered her sympathies and inquired as to what she could do to prepare for my arrival. I mechanically told her to contact my daughter and that I would get back to her.

As I hung up the phone, my business manager happened to be standing right beside me. The look in my eyes prompted him to ask the nature of the phone call. It was as if someone else were speaking but the words were coming out of my mouth; my mother just died. He looked as if an action was required and turned and gave the message to a friend standing nearby. She went down to the birthday celebrations and informed my Teacher of this news. She outlined some quick instructions. Get a plane ticket, get a car to drive her to the airport, someone go pack her things, bring her luggage here, and bring her to me. These instructions were filled with lightning speed.

I sat in front of my Teacher, who encouraged me to talk about my mother. I could sense being filled with an enormous amount of strength and courage as she talked with me. She said for me to do a certain prayer for myself as I was driven to the airport. Then, on the plane, do the prayer for my mother. She also said to let my dad and brothers take complete charge of the funeral; for me to just attend as a guest. It was good that this was said, because my family had planned on excluding me from the services anyway. They were more than a little upset that the December funeral plans had radically changed. They had so much to explain to their friends. This weird sister with this strange healing power had extended mother's life for four months.

My mother came to me quite often in the next few weeks. I was not quite so excited to see her. Sometimes I was just a little afraid of "the other side." The other side is always fascinating. If a message needs to be delivered a way will be found. One afternoon, I "saw" a golden chariot with large shiny wheels drive into my living room. A grand warrior was driving and a goddess, with jeweled, braided hair, sat right beside him. The chariot came to an abrupt halt as the goddess stepped out and started walking toward me. I was transfixed. It was like a dream. As the goddess came closer to me, her white goddess gown fell away to reveal a suit I quickly recognized as one my mother wore! Then, I looked up at the goddesses' face; the face and hair had completely changed into my mother's face and hairstyle, right down to her glasses.

In my surprised state, my mother wasted no time. She had used a safe ploy to enter my space without frightening me. She had little time in the earth vibration and was determined to get her message to me. She sat beside me and began to talk. She talked of my childhood, some troubled times, about the karma that I had accepted for this lifetime, and how the karma had been distorted and expanded. She explained that sometimes there are accidents and the plan can change. She was apologizing for some actions over which she felt responsibility. I was not given any space in which to engage with her. I somehow knew I could not touch her, that there would be nothing to touch.

However, I could clearly see and hear her.

I soon went back to New York. I love New York. There is a temple in which I enjoy sitting and meditating. In this temple I asked God how my mother was and what was she doing. A vision of sorts appeared and I saw my mother in school, studying very hard. I asked the meaning of this vision. The answer was that she would soon return in another body and was studying to learn her role and her script for the next life on earth.

She is back, in the form of my first grandchild, born four years after my mother left us. It has been clear from the moment this child took her first breath as to who she was. My mother's hands were slightly deformed. She could type and play the piano, but physically there was a lack of perfection, so to speak. My granddaughter, from just a few days old, would bring her hands in front of her face and examine them. She would turn them around, wave them back and forth, hold them away from her and then bring them close to her. Intuitively I understood that she was delighting in perfectly formed hands. Many other actions since then have revealed how special her hands are to her. Wanting more proof, I asked my daughter to send a photo of my granddaughter to me. My granddaughter has a very unusual Welsh name, as did my mother! When the photo was taken, they just happened to be standing by a village sign. The sign had my mother's name, then my granddaughter's name, side by side. And, the photo was taken on a vacation in Wales.

Kevin

A few years back, Kevin, at age thirteen, was diagnosed with a very aggressive brain cancer. The doctors said that he would be blind in two weeks and dead in one month. The parents, in shock, raced to a psychologist for assistance in dealing with the emotional aspects of this information. The psychologist was a client of mine and immediately telephoned to tell me that he was sending this family to see me.

About an hour later the doorbell rang. The mother, father and son, stunned and dismayed, walked into my Reiki office.

They were quick to tell me that they were only in my office at the encouragement of the psychologist and did not know about or necessarily believe in what I did. This is common conversation for me. I invited them in, offered them some refreshment and we chatted for a while. Kevin was silent. The mother talked most of the time, with the father interjecting now and then. I explained a little of what I did and what I would do that day. And, we would take it a day at a time.

After requesting that the parents observe in silence, I invited Kevin to lie on his back on my treatment table. I made him comfortable with pillows for his head, under his knees and a light blanket over his body. I then positioned my chair at his head. I rested my elbows on a wedge-type pillow in my lap so only the weight of my hands would rest on his head. I placed a tissue over his eyes so he would not be bothered by any light and also to assist him in relaxing. After this was all done I placed my hands, palms down, on the top of his head. I left them there for about fifteen minutes. The next placement was over his eyes for another fifteen minutes, followed by a placement over his ears for the same length of time. I then stood at his right side and placed both my hands, palms down, over his solar plexus area. This is the emotional power center and my hand reactions will inform me of existing energy changes there.

At the end of the hour I was able to tell them the size, location and description of Kevin's tumor. It was exactly as the tests had revealed. My next requirement was to initiate the entire family into the basic level of Reiki Touch Therapy so the energy of Reiki could be maintained in between treatments with me. The compassionate atmosphere of Reiki had calmed them and a trust level was established. I initiated the three of them, appointments were made for future visits, and they left. Part of the initiation instruction was to have everyone do Reiki Touch Therapy on Kevin every day.

From that moment on Kevin got up and went to bed an hour early so he could do Reiki on himself. The mother and father alternated times but added another two hours each day between them. Within a week, Kevin's vision had returned to normal, he was back in school and had caught up with all his homework. At school he would lean onto one hand and do Reiki at his desk in the classroom. Within a month he was trying out for the baseball team and his coveted spot of shortstop.

My general schedule for one with cancer is a twenty-one-day treatment plan. Everyday, for twenty-one days. During this time, with the aid of crystals, etheric surgery procedures and skill, I performed several "brain surgeries" on Kevin. One of his parents always accompanied his sessions. One day I remarked that even though the tumor was shrinking in size there were several tentacles projecting from the baseball size tumor. They confirmed that had also been detected with the MRI. One particular shape of crystal has a "sliced" or slanted terminal point. This is the type I use for surgery. A crystal can be programmed to etherically enter an area and do what you direct it to do. Two of my crystals are encased in silver with a small handle. It becomes, as such, a scalpel. After about a half hour of Reiki, during which I communicate with the tumor, the tentacles and the bone and brain around it, I enter the etheric space. The etheric space is the area just outside of the physical, dense energy form. This space has a quick energy, allowing one to move through it without any obstacles. Everything in the physical is contained within the etheric body, except the density.

With intense focus I pointed the tip of the crystal toward the connection of the tentacle on the tumor. Carefully, with compassion, I informed the tumor that the tentacles are compromising the function of Kevin's brain. The tumor surrendered the tentacles as the scalpel gently severed the connection. One by one, sometimes reluctantly giving up their territory, the tentacles came off. I guided these out of the brain, through the skull, up into the air where an angel was waiting with open hands. The angel took the tentacles to a place where they could be happy without harming anyone. The Reiki Touch Therapy, slowly but surely, shrunk Kevin's tumor and it was gone. Kevin was fourteen.

Kevin recovered quickly. The doctors sat around a conference table and could only claim it as a miracle. He had received no chemotherapy, no radiation and no surgery. Kevin was accepted into an exclusive private school and again tried out and got his coveted shortstop position on the baseball team. After his freshman year and into his sophomore year Kevin's parents began to have marital problems. Kevin's illness had taken a toll on the relationship and home atmosphere. Kevin felt responsible, began to have bouts of depression and his appetite faltered. Teenage boys do not usually have appetite problems!

The tense home atmosphere accelerated and Kevin seemed to absorb the anxiety like a sponge. He began to get nauseated and to have headaches. His ability on the baseball field was faltering. He was disoriented. They returned to the cancer center for tests. Kevin's tumor had returned. In the hospital room the doctor was outlining the chemotherapy and radiation schedule. The tumor was aggressive, large and inoperable. Kevin asked the doctors if this treatment was going to cure him. The doctors said that due to the rapid progression of the tumor that it would not but it was the only thing they knew to do. Kevin threw back the hospital bed sheets, hopped out of bed and stated that he knew something else to do—Reiki. Kevin was now into his sixteenth year.

Kevin had not had Reiki Touch Therapy treatments with me for a couple of years. To our knowledge there was no need. Now there was. We renewed the treatments. Kevin's parents also talked him into radiation treatments and steroids. The Reiki seemed to reinstate his ability to stay in school, but the baseball effort was thwarted. However, a really cute girlfriend balanced that out. She made Kevin very happy.

The parents continued to pursue separate lives. The question of custody came up and Kevin was again thrown into a fear of whom he would be with. Mom wanted him to be her little boy and Dad wanted him to be his young man. Kevin was torn, but wanted to be with his dad. Court times were scheduled; the tension was high. Kevin's mother hired an independent neurologist to testify that because of Kevin's brain cancer, he was unable to make coherent and stable decisions. Kevin ended up with his mother.

He became sicker and had to drop out of school. The pain, growth of the tumor, the depression and disorientation were all taking Kevin's life force away from him. We spoke often on the phone. He wanted to know about dying. We talked about what all he had done with his short life. I asked him if there was something he wanted to do that he had not done. One thing was to attend a professional baseball game during the World Series. The *Make a Wish* organization fulfilled Kevin's dream and flew him to San Francisco for a game. He was accompanied by a well-known sports personality who was able to get Kevin a seat in the dugout with the players. He returned with a baseball signed by all his favorite players. Kevin personally experienced his field of dreams.

Just as he was consciously realizing that his life was ending his body was compensating for that realization. Kevin went into a coma and returned to the hospital. He passed away into his field of baseball dreams at age sixteen and a half.

There was a terrific thunderstorm on the day of his funeral. During the ceremony a large tree, a landmark for that church, was struck by lightning, split in two and burst into flames. The tree completely burned to the ground.

A few days later Kevin's mother called me and asked if I would like to accompany her to Kevin's gravesite. Of course I would. I thought that I should rush out and buy all kinds of flowers for the grave. Something stopped me. I sat and meditated. I asked Kevin what he wanted. He described everything to me in detail. I was to get several silver bowls. One was to contain holy water, another some jasmine rice which had particular spices in it, another some sacred ash, and others for specific flower petals. There were prayers and chants to be done to infuse these items with love, peace, grace and good wishes for his journey onward. I went out and obtained these items and spent the evening in preparation.

The next morning Kevin's mom drove into my driveway and honked to announce her arrival. My hands were full and I made two trips from my house to her car. She quizzically threw me a look, but said nothing. I did not explain. We drove to the site. A light rain began from a perfect blue sky.

We thought nothing of it. At the cemetery we walked a short distance to his gravesite. She had a potted plant and placed it where the headstone would soon be. After standing in silence I told her that I brought a few things and had a ceremony to perform if I had her permission. Actually, I already had Kevin's permission but it was polite to ask. She was extremely curious and quickly agreed.

I asked her to help bring the items from the car. There was a silver tray, the silver bowls, a glass bottle of holy water, sacred ash, rice and flower petals, all in separate closed containers. We put them down a couple of feet from his grave and I began to prepare everything in the silver bowls. I was chanting softly. The chants were for blessings, to remove obstacles and for his protection on his continuing journey. We had not noticed that the sky had become totally black. All of a sudden an explosive thunderclap filled the air, followed by a torrent of huge raindrops pelting down upon us. Kevin's mom wanted to race back to the car, but I knew it was the heavens acknowledging and supporting the blessings. She stayed. As the appropriate Mantras were chanted I said Kevin's name, his age and his earthly location. I put a handful of the special, blessed rice where his crown chakra, the top of his head, was resting. Going on down, I placed a handful of rice at his third eye, throat, heart, solar and sacral plexus and the root chakra at the base of his spine. I then placed the holy rice at his hands, knees and feet. Following, in the same order, I sprinkled the holy water over each little mound of rice, all the while chanting the appropriate Mantras. His mother was unfamiliar with these and was silent and reverent as I did the ritual for her son. The last part was to scatter flower petals over the entire site. It was sweet and very colorful. The thunder was deafening and the lightning was bright. We were drenched by the stinging, pelting rain, but did not notice. We knew it was for Kevin and we were not in any danger.

After I poured the rest of the rice and the holy water around the perimeter of his grave, we stood and silently paid our respects to this incredibly brave young man. I am sure we both honored his strength, as well as his fortitude, during his illness. He was a warrior battling his cancer; a hero continuing to live life to the fullest during pain and sorrow. He got his last wish of attending his favorite team's baseball game. All in all, even though a tear trickled down his cheek as he took his last earthly breath, I believe he died content. He lived a greater and more fulfilling life than many ninety-year-old folks.

Andy

In 1983 I was traveling and studying holistic medical techniques in the Orient. Upon my return, my mother telephoned to inform me that I had a new nephew. I was delighted and inquired as to his name, weight and the reactions of the family. My mother answered my questions, and then there was a long pause. I sensed something but did not know what. Mother began to cry and said that something was wrong with the baby—he was diagnosed with Down Syndrome. The family had known that there was a possibility of an abnormality with this birth. His mother was in her forties and had colon cancer. The pregnancy was difficult at best.

Other than the Down Syndrome, all his vitals were fine. He was very tiny, weighing less than five pounds. My brother has a doctoral degree in psychology and felt very able to care for his son. He was named after another brother of mine, Andy, and was a very welcome baby.

It was very difficult for mother to discuss Andy's diagnosis. I could tell that she had projected into the already happening future and knew she would be the baby's primary caregiver. It was actually only a few months before his mother passed away, and my mother moved in to care for Andy and his older sister until my brother remarried two years later.

That same evening after the call, I was meditating, naturally having my sweet, new nephew on my mind. I was "imagining" him in his crib at home. He was now seven days old. I "imagined" the decorations in the nursery and felt comfortable that he was loved and cared for. As the meditation progressed I astrally traveled to an area above his home and could see the roof. Suddenly a beautiful angel appeared and floated down to the roof just above Andy's crib. She pointed her finger and flames darted out onto the roof. A hole, large enough for the angel, was created and she entered the home. I saw her pick Andy up into her arms, give him a hug and an angelic smile, and float back up out of the roof.

She continued to rise up above Andy's home and the neighborhood. I was straining my eyes to keep them in sight. Then, she looked down at me, and with her head, motioned for me to accompany them. We flew through many constellations of stars, beautiful moons and planets for what seemed a very long time. She motioned to a planet and indicated that it was where we were going. I silently followed her, realizing I was a guest and observer. I was grateful to be invited.

The angel, carefully cradling Andy in her loving arms, knew exactly where she was going. A building appeared and she entered it through the roof (no flames this time). A group of "doctors" were waiting for her. Now, these doctors were not in human form. The heads were very large, the bodies were very small. There were slits for eyes and I saw no mouth. The arms were long and slim, as were the hands. The seven doctors were surrounding a long aluminum-type table. Andy was handed to them and placed on the center of the table. The communication between the doctors was nonverbal. The angel and I hovered above and to the side and waited for them to work with Andy.

Soon the technique was decided, as well as to which doctors would do the procedure. Some of the doctors took one step back. One doctor handed another doctor a paper-thin metal strip, about three or four inches long. This strip was silver in color and had some embossed, or raised, Braille-like dots. Andy was lying very still on the table. A bright, but also soft, silvery glowlight was above him. It had x-ray capabilities, which I found curious because the angel informed me that the doctors also had this capability. The doctor holding the metal strip held it above Andy's forehead. He gently laid it horizontally on his head. As the doctor placed it, he moved back and watched as the metal was absorbed into Andy's head.

The doctors conferred again and another doctor stepped forward as the previous doctor stepped back one step. A longer piece of metal was handed to this new doctor. It was about seven or eight inches in length and also had the raised bumps on it. The doctor held the metal strip vertically above the center of Andy's tiny torso. Slowly, with all the doctors lending focused energy, he lowered the metal onto the pink skin and it was absorbed into the baby's torso. Now, all the doctors stepped forward. The focus was indeed, and appropriately, heavenly. The doctors' long slim arms and hands stretched out from around the treatment table over Andy's little body. Andy had remained perfectly still, with his eyes closed, the entire time. A soft, pastel light emanated from the doctors' hands, and the area where the third eye would be had a more focused red light sweeping the body. They seemed to stand there for a long time.

I do not know how long the entire procedure lasted.

The light from the doctor's hands and third eye seemed to pull back into their forms. In unison the doctors took three steps back and bowed their heads. After a while they looked up at the angel and motioned that their work was done and she could have the infant. The angel went to each doctor and smiled a magnificent smile of gratitude, then picked up the baby, motioned to me, and off we went.

The trip back was as spectacular as the trip there. Finding doctors on another planet and seeing the procedures done on my nephew was amazing in and of itself. I knew I could tell few, if any, people about this experience! Andy was awake now and his eyes were taking in the sparkling light of the stars. He seemed like an older, more mature baby, not one just seven days old. There was a different energy about him. He was actively moving around so he could observe and enjoy this journey.

The angel seemed to think this was normal behavior and was surprised that I was surprised. Now, think about it . . . how could anyone not be surprised by the entire adventure!

We arrived back at the opening in the roof just over Andy's nursery. The house was silent and everyone was sleeping soundly.

The exquisite angel gently put Andy back into his crib. He did not want her to go. He wanted to play! He was laughing and waving his arms and legs about. I thought that was most unusual, but so was the evening. The angel came up out of the roof, again produced flames out of her fingers, which this time closed and sealed the roof. She looked at me in an assessing kind of way, and saw that I would adjust and be all right with this experience. With an angelic smile she spread her wings and lifted up and became part of the spectacular night sky.

I came out of meditation and thought, "wow, what a trip!" Normally, one is peaceful and serene after meditation, but this time I was exhausted and fell sound asleep.

The next evening my mother called and was talking so fast I had to ask her to slow down because I could not follow what she was saying. She said that that morning Andy had held his head up and had shown signs that he recognized family members. She said that he was very active, happy and was not at all acting like an infant with Down Syndrome. My mother had, I am sure, secretly hoped that the doctors had made a mistake with her first grandson, and that he did not really have a mental challenge after all. She was very excited. The whole family was. My brother decided not to go to work that day and to call the hospital and request that Andy be retested. After hearing about Andy's activities the doctors were agreeable to that.

The doctors were puzzled. The tests immediately after birth definitely showed a full spectrum of Down Syndrome. But, now, eight days later, this seemed like a different child altogether. He was lifting his head, turning over and had an upper torso strength remarkable for this situation and for his age. The final conclusion was that Andy was not as severely delayed as first diagnosed; that he was "borderline."

Mother was ecstatically relating the day's activities to me. I was ecstatically listening and thrilled, too. At that moment I had no memory of the previous meditation experience.

As time and years passed, Andy seemed to have capabilities in certain areas, ordinarily out of his range of ability. He was almost a genius with anything electronic. At age two he could work with any computer. The remote control for the television was child's play. The video games at the arcades were also simple. He was especially drawn to those that had a space motif. If an older boy, even a teenager, was playing one of the video games, my brother would hold Andy up to the screen and Andy would tell the boy, "this way, now that way." The older boys were astounded that this disabled toddler knew more than they did.

Andy is now twenty years old. He attended a regular public school and did very well, especially in technical arenas. Being very wise, his father chose not to have any corrective surgeries on him. He knew that Andy had come to the family as a very special boy. He wanted Andy to acknowledge his karma and to live the life he chose. My brother became and still is, a very active individual for programs for all mentally challenged children. Even when Andy was a few months old he would take him to his Rotary Club and Kiwanis Club meetings. He would hand his son to the first man on the first row. He instructed him to hold Andy, to communicate with him, then pass him on to the next person, until everyone in the room had held his son. As my brother would lead the program he would tell the audience that all children were part of the world, that all children deserved to be in the world and not hidden because they were different. He said, "This is my son and this is your neighbor and this is your community, which will serve these children." And, they do.

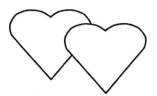

THROAT
Gabrielle

E ven though the throat is an important area of the body I have had few clients with throat problems. I will share the processes and procedures employed with this situation.

The throat is home to our fifth chakra and the aura of the throat is blue. If an individual has an expanded blue aura, they are more than likely a singer, teacher, newscaster or a professional speaker of some sort. Overuse of the throat, lack of rest of the vocal cords, or exposure to respiratory problems can result in colds or laryngitis.

If one has an imbalance or discomfort in the throat it is usually considered common sense to drink plenty of liquids and to monitor any speaking activities.

Once in a while I will have a client in my office with a throat imbalance. They instruct me to do energy work on the throat. With ordinary Reiki practice I do not put my hands on or near the vocal cords or the windpipe area because it could bring up hidden or suppressed traumas. Notice that some people will not wear tight ties, turtleneck sweaters or scarves closed around the throat. My thinking is that these individuals, for some reason, have a fear of their breath being taken away, or seriously compromised in some way. It could be in this lifetime; a severe throat imbalance; or possibly the client lost their head in a previous life experience. Many punishments were meted out in the form of "off with his head" activities. Unless the client specifically insists that I touch his or her throat, I do not.

I will counsel a client either over the phone or in person and use a guided imagery technique. This is usually having the client imagine that they are drinking a warm, healing liquid. Most of the time this is an emerald green, liquid Reiki drink. The Reiki drink brings balance and harmony to the body, mind and soul. Frequently I will have them imagine that they are drinking a warm, golden nectar. An image is created so the golden drink is absorbed into the painful or problematic area. This can be done by the client without me, but we all, when we are not feeling well, want the comfort of a practitioner for support.

One professional speaker was having chronic sore throats. Her job was to speak, often and for a long period of time. I did a lot of distance energy focusing as she was too far away for hands on treatment. I had her drink the warm, liquid Reiki drink, as well as the golden nectar. This was all on an etheric level, of course. I could sense the panic in the speaker and all who promoted her. One evening I decided to "call in the troops." Now, who are the troops? The troops are those you deem to be a higher power you can call on to assist when you think your work is insufficient.

The troops assisted me in placing two shawls on a large, flat surface—one red and one white. The red was for energy and the white for purity. I did a protection method around this area, which I will call an altar. The protection method was to seal in the area. I had four crystals that I placed at each corner, with the point, or terminus, of the crystal, pointing inward toward the center. The crystals were for focus. I lit candles for the "flickering tongues of angels." I bowed and honored all ten directions. On a pretty piece of paper, pink in color, I drew, as best I could, the client's throat. I placed this paper in the center of the two shawls, half on the red one and half on the white. I endeavored to psychically enter the throat to explore and discover the imbalance. There was a red patch which seemed to be covering another, larger red patch, and even another. Also apparent were other, smaller patches about to surface.

The troops were standing around the altar, in readiness for "battle." St. Michael was there with his sword and used it to cut out the imbalances, all of them, in the throat. As the imbalances were cut out, a group of healers were present to provide the appropriate energies for a thorough and complete healing. A choir of angels chanted to appease and calm the process. Other angels provided light, color and more energy. I placed my hands on the drawing and empowered the throat to be forever and always healed and available for its owner.

I did a meditation and asked the throat what its purpose was in this lifetime. I asked the throat what it needed from its owner to be healed and to function in the needed capacity. The purpose was to share the word of God and the need was gratitude. I asked the owner to express, in her own way, gratitude for the work her throat did for her. I asked the owner to give her throat a gift along with a promise that gratitude would always be present. I asked the throat to continue with its work, knowing that gratitude would always be present. At the end of the process a sense of completion occurred. It was as if all parties had an instant notification that the work was done and that it was a success.

To my knowledge the throat is fine. I do know that the speaker has continued her talks and her voice is powerful and pure. Thank you, God.

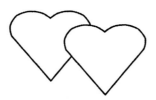

EYES, EARS and MORE
Dan

The ringing of the phone challenged the reverie of a beautiful spring day. It was the husband of another client of mine—a husband who had not been supportive of these fringe medicine-healing arts. However, this time it was he who had an emergency. If this was not handled properly he could be blind in a very short time. At the moment it was just one eye involved but an ophthalmologist assured him that it would indeed spread to the other eye.

Dan nervously entered my office. I think he expected to see skulls on the walls, or to smell incense. The office was professional, clean, serene and welcoming. He relaxed a tiny bit.

I offered him some water or juice or tea. That act alone surprised him. I might be human after all. However, he did not accept it. I asked him to tell me what the doctor's diagnosis and plan of treatment was.

His words tumbled out of his mouth, incongruous and not in sequence. I took notes and read them back to him. After a while a picture of the situation developed. Dan's right eye membrane was deteriorating and fluid was seeping through this membrane. The prognosis was a loss of direct vision and the physician advised emergency surgery. Dan chose to see me first. He came for three one-hour sessions three days in a row. In addition to the Reiki Touch Therapy I advised no television, no reading, some positive thinking affirmations and some breathing exercises. The unusual part was using a folk remedy of one teaspoon of milk placed on a cotton pad, taped to his eye and left on overnight. What did he have to lose? What did he have to gain? Sight.

Dan followed all the instructions to the letter. On the fourth day he was seen by his physician who thought it was the other eye and not the one at risk. After that was cleared up the doctor asked him to return in a week. We did more Reiki sessions and Dan did more milk infused cotton pads. At the next appointment the doctor couldn't explain this amazing turn of events, but advised Dan to return again for a checkup in one month. At that appointment Dan's eye was perfectly clear, the membrane was intact and secure and no lymphatic fluid was seeping through. After twenty years the eyes are still just fine.

Jo

This is a combination of ears, eyes, head and heart. Jo has a congenital hearing disorder, has worn glasses for most of her life, and has headaches and a congenital heart murmur.

At the time I saw her I was combining acupressure and Reiki Touch Therapy in the same session. I thought perhaps that the acupressure would open some energy lines and then the Reiki would balance them out. You will observe the illustrations of the acupressure points for the mentioned imbalances. After a half hour of acupressure on all the points another half hour of Reiki would be applied. I did this procedure on many patients. The end result was that I discovered two things. One, the Reiki did it all. Two, the individual who came for Reiki did not want to be prodded and pushed. Reiki is a gentle, patterned touch over clothing and the addition of acupressure soon became incongruous for me. Reiki will get to the source, or the cause, of all imbalances.

In a later letter to me Jo stated that in addition to a solution for her headaches, ear and eye problems, a real shift in her attitude and consciousness had occurred, as well as an overall approval of life. She further stated that her entire family had significantly benefited from Reiki and the Reiki clinics held each week.

There are many acupressure books and some differences occur within each one. The meridian lines of energy are addressed in acupressure, as well as acupuncture. A needle can more accurately target an area than the tip of a finger. Some individuals are uncomfortable with needles so the acupressure serves them well. The following drawings are the acupressure points used on Jo and Dan for their ears, eyes, head and heart. Some others are for energy and for circulation.

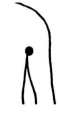

Left armpit deep
Arterial circulation

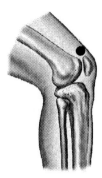

Soft tissue above
patella
Heart, lymph

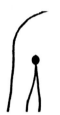

Right armpit deep
Veinous circulation

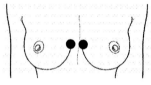

Sternum & breast muscle
Ears - deafness

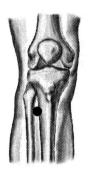

Bifurcation of
tibia & fibula
Heart, lymph

Apply simultaneously
Eyestrain - headache

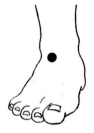

Ankle - between
ankle & tibia at
foot - soft spot
Eyes

Apply simultaneously
Mid-forhead - eyes

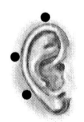

Mastoid & ears

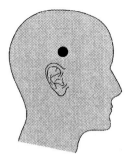

Just below sylvian fissure - where
parietal meets frontal - Headache

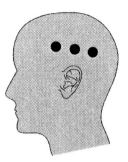

Left sylvian fissure Capillaries
of heart & lungs

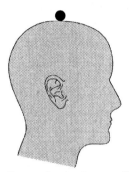

Directly on fonanelle (soft spot)
Headache

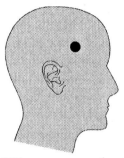

Where temporal joins frontal
Eyes & ears

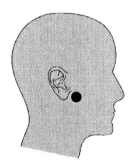

Under jaw bone in
front of ear
Heart

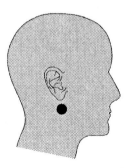

Posterior jaw bone under ear -
pull forward
Eyes

A Memorium
Eternal Vision

They know me not, who think that I am

only flesh and blood. . .

A transient dweller on this fragile spaceship earth

that gave me human birth.

For I am spirit eternal, indestructible, not confined to space or time

and when my sojourn here is through, my roles fulfilled,

my assignments done,

I will lay aside this spacesuit called my body and move on to other mansions, roles, assignments in our father's house of eternal life.

So, do dry your tears, weep not overmuch for me - or for yourself.

Set me free, in the love that holds us all and makes us one eternally!

Our paths will cross again, our minds and hearts will touch.

Our souls will shout with joy and laughter as we recall the lives we've lived, the worlds we've seen, the ways we've trod

to find ourselves—at last—in God.

J. Sig Paulson

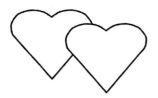

HEART
Sig

I knew the day before, as did he. I allowed myself no external planning, and advanced no preparation; just remained open to my cosmic guidance. He was grey in color and moving slowly to accommodate his state.

When he was comfortable on my healing table, my guides began to instruct me, "Loosen up the body, gently, head to toe, for relaxation and to open up the energy avenues." I made the comment that he had been out of his body a lot lately and asked him how it was. He just smiled.

As his chest was massaged, a great deal of energy formed; alive and electric. I was guided to get my crystal. With the heart area as a focal point, I used the crystal to open the arteries and veins all over his body, head to toe. Subclavian, aorta, coronary, femoral, carotid, jugular and others were opened. The valves of his heart were open wide and life was freely flowing throughout his body. I pressed firmly and deeply on and around the heart, inhaling and exhaling to the rhythm.

I assisted him in sitting up and I synchronized the pressure from behind and in front of the heart. I energized this area with all my strength. I assisted him in resuming his supine position on the treatment table. I noticed my hands becoming rigid. Into the etheric body they went. With my fingers pointed, like a scalpel, they separated the sides of the heart, the top of the heart, and the bottom portion from the rest of the body. Just as I was about to go deeper I was stopped. Dr. Forrest, Dr. Murphy and Dr. Brown, doctors in spirit, appeared.

Many times with etheric surgery, and also other shamanistic procedures, spirit entities will come in and either do the surgery themselves or instruct me how or both. This time they chose to have me observe. I stood back and watched as they clamped off the main arteries and quickly removed a greatly enlarged heart. Just as quickly they secured a smaller, energized, pumping heart. The clamps were removed and the arteries and veins reconnected. They proceeded with much haste to wrap the heart in an etheric, mistlike material; an etheric bandage.

The doctors in spirit nodded for me to step in to the body area again. I was instructed to do Reiki Touch Therapy to balance and harmonize the new organ with the rest of his body. My deepest honor.

I thanked them and went to work. It did not take long to balance. The doctors were very skilled and thorough with their work and his body was so grateful and accepting of the new organ.

I was guided to go to his head to scan the entire body. There were other problems to address, but not for that day. I was then guided to do the "Chalice" technique, learned from Jean Houston, PhD Standing beside the solar plexus I very slowly raised my hands. My body becomes the Chalice stem and base. As my hands rise into the air, I call upon my guides, my spiritual masters and teachers. These are many. My Guru, the ascended Reiki Masters, Usui, Hayashi and Takata, Mother Mary, Quan Yin, St. Germain, Thoth, Drs. Forrest, Murphy and Brown, holy angels and saints and departed known healers. I ask their aid in filling my "Chalice" with all that they are and all that I am. Music, floral scents, wisdom, power, knowledge, information—all filled the Chalice. I am that I am. My Chalice is full to the brim. As I bow toward my client's body I bless, endow and empower his being with the contents of the Chalice, all that I am, and all that he is.

The Chalice empties slowly into his being, penetrating and permeating the surgery section, and further, into every cell of his body. The flow is tangible as it fills and balances throughout. It is now all out of the Chalice and into his body. My hands lift and meet in a prayer position, touching the all-knowing third eye.

I gently and slowly back out of his aura space, bowing the entire time and repeating, "I am as I am." I must acknowledge and give gratitude to the "I am" to remain full, to give it away as needed. Now, after this etheric surgery his aura was such a bright green that I could have backed out of the entire building. But, of course, I stayed with him. After a period of time I opened my eyes and took another deep breath of gratitude. The spirit doctors had gone. After a few moments his eyes opened. Neither of us spoke.

After a while, I stepped close to him and softly said, "You have a new heart." "I know," he said. I told him it was up to him to interpret what a "new heart" meant to him and for him to take that information to use for his future. It could be physical with renewed energy; it could be the loving, nurturing nature of the heart; it could be a combination and also many other "heart opening" ideas. He went on, continuing to spread love and light, with great energy for a number of years. His name is mentioned very often, with great respect and admiration.

Andreè

Over twenty years ago a petite, middle-aged lady from England came to hear a Reiki lecture. During the lecture I walked around, fielding questions, putting my hands on people's shoulders or heads for a minute or two. After the lecture the English lady came over to me and said that she had suffered from back pain for many years and now, with only a minute or two of Reiki, it was gone. She went on to say that she had a grown daughter with a severe heart and lung problem and asked if I would see her.

Over the next week or so I met and treated her daughter Andreè. She had been born and raised in England, was married, had a toddler, and lived in Houston, Texas. Before the Reiki sessions Andreè's hands and feet were cyanotic, or blue. They were also somewhat atrophied due to lack of circulation and activity. She could not stand for over twenty minutes, could not pick up and carry her two-year-old child, and her legs would collapse if she tried to make up her bed or do any ordinary housework.

Many readers will have heard of Texas Children's Hospital and of David, the "bubble boy." David was in a protective plastic "room" for his entire life, due to an immune imbalance. Well, Andreè was in the "bubble" next to David. However, she did not have the severity of the disorder and was able to be at home and live a somewhat normal life. She had an open heart valve and just one lung.

After five Reiki Touch Therapy sessions, Andreè started hitting tennis balls with her husband. This evolved into regularly playing nine holes of golf with friends. In addition to the Reiki I taught her to meditate and to do visual imagery for putting affirmations into her body, mind and spirit. Soon, she was able to lift and carry her child and participate in her school activities. Andree` also became active in her church, doing volunteer charity work for the homeless. Andreè was fiery and political in this endeavor. Indeed, she was, for the first time in her life, living a completely normal and active life. She continued her Reiki treatments and furthered her Reiki training, as well.

Years later, Andreè's mother was in town and we all went out to lunch. Andreè and I had the same birthday so we felt connected to each other in a unique way. She felt I had saved her life. I was grateful for the Reiki! At lunch I noticed a pager attached to Andreè's waist. I casually remarked as to how popular she had become being on call! I noticed Andreè's mother getting very quiet and staring down at her food. Andreè informed me that the pager was to notify her when a heart-lung match donor was found for her. She wanted to have a new heart and a new lung to improve her life even more. I looked at her and realized that she had just spelled out her death plan. She knew it, too. We were all silent in that knowing.

Six months later Andreè telephoned me and in an excited voice said that a donor had been found and she was on her way to the hospital for the transplant surgery. My prayers had been, honestly, that no donor would ever be found. Her mother and dad flew over from England to be with their only daughter. I was there, along with her husband and her now eight-year-old child. Hope was the only way any of us could get through this so "hope" became our mantra. The surgery went well. Andreè progressed beautifully for three weeks. She was about to go home with very frequent rehabilitation follow-up schedule but she developed a stomach ulcer. It did not seem too serious, but it was an infection, so the hospital stay was lengthened a bit. We minimized it and firmly held on to our mantra, "hope." She was dressed in new finery and happily bouncing around in her hospital room.

When the ulcer was under control enough to make plans to go home, we were all very elated and much relieved. Then she caught a cold. A respiratory infection with a new lung—not a reassuring sign. We again dove into our "hope" mantra. As we involved ourselves with the tedious medical explanations, we endeavored to understand any words that would equate to our mantra, "hope." Andreè's spirits were remarkable. Each little symptom was a minor setback, just a normal occurrence for a surgery like this. It was a day-to-day schedule with a calendar clearly marked "home." We did not comment on the constantly changing dates.

The lung collapsed. It was being rejected by the body's immune system. With that the heart was in jeopardy also. The doctors told the family to expect the worst. Her parents leaned very heavily on me. I had, according to them, accomplished one miracle after another with Andreè, why not another? Andreè's mother also went into her comatose daughter's critical care unit and told her how strong she was, how much she had to live for, how young she was and that all of life was in front of her. Even though I was not a member of the family the doctors allowed me to go in. I had asked for a particular ancient chant, known to produce miracles, to be played in her room. Due to all the electrical machines the chant had to be on a battery-operated recorder. However, even just the sound of this chant would cause her blood pressure to rise, her pulses to race and produce great agitation in Andreè. I was disappointed but the doctors said it had to go.

One evening, at about eight o'clock, I went into the unit. Andreè's eyes and mouth were fixed wide open. This is common in the last stages. There were wires and tubes attached to virtually all parts of her body, including every finger. I searched for a space in which to put one hand in place to perform Reiki on her. There wasn't one. Finally I put a few fingers on top of her head. I softly began to chant an ancient Mantra. In a few seconds her eyes and mouth relaxed and gently closed. The hospital had called her minister. He came to see her but when he approached her unit there was such a bright light coming out of the room, he could not see her, or me, or a bed, or any machines. The minister brought the nurse, who also witnessed this phenomenon.

I knew that it was time for Andreè to go. I also knew that her mother was not about to let her go. I spoke to Andreè and told her that it was her life. She had lived a life of many trials and she could do whatever she needed and wanted to do. I saw a slight smile. I continued. I told her that her husband and child would be just fine. I said that her parents would also be all right, too. Then, I said, "Andreè, you have to show your mother a sign that it is time for her to let you go. You must do something so it will be clear that you must now go. It was eight-fifteen in the evening.

The nurse and the minister were standing outside the unit, still blinded by the light. I asked them to go and get both parents, her husband and her child. As they all entered and stood by Andreè's bed, I kissed the top of her head and whispered, "Goodbye, my dear friend, I will always remember your courage." At that moment a trickle of blood began to seep out the side of Andreè's mouth. Her mother exclaimed, "Oh, Andreè, you have suffered too much! Please, I do not want you to suffer more, you must go to God." Within about ten minutes Andreè took an audible and deep breath, how we do not know, with no functioning lung at all, and left her body. It was eight-thirty in the evening, very near her birthday in April.

The church was filled for her services. Yellow roses were everywhere. Members of the church, neighbors and community members praised her civic accomplishments. Andreè left a legacy of courage for all to witness.

Gemma

Adiary account of a three-year-old heart patient, written by her mother. It relates traditional medicine, Reiki Touch Therapy and her shared spiritual path.

On June 9, at a routine exam, Rose Lee, the nurse practitioner that we were seeing as a family practitioner discovered a heart murmur that she found disturbing. She had Ted, the doctor, come down and have a listen. He sent us to Children's Hospital. On June 16 (your grandparent's anniversary), an echocardiogram was done to see what was going on.

We realized that something was wrong when the technicians would not talk to us. They were kind of pointing things out to each other on the screen. You watched a Barney video and were pretty calm about all of this—just accepting it. There was no pain involved but occasionally your lip would quiver and reveal your anxiety—or perhaps reflect ours.

After a long and anxious hour in the waiting area, the doctors finally came to get us. They told us that you had two holes in your heart—in the septal wall between the atria and a cleft (tear) in the mitral valve. There is also a slightly narrowed aorta, but there is nothing they feel they need to do about that. In order to repair the holes and the valve, you need open heart surgery.

We were stunned. Your Dad had to leave the room so that you would not see how upset he was. While one doctor talked to us, you played with the other one—almost as though you were trying to separate yourself from our talk. I am sure that you sensed something was wrong, but we didn't tell you anything. We met with child psychologists at the hospital and they all said not to tell you until a few days before. I am afraid that we listened to them—not considering enough the fact that you would feel our anxiety and sadness at what was to come.

The surgery was scheduled for August 3. It was so hard for me to even pick a date. I went for long walks trying to choose between August 1 or 8. Then settled on the third. We wanted to do it as quickly as possible. The third gave me time to wrap up my work and take you on vacation for two and a half weeks. There was to be a meditation intensive on July 30 entitled the "Blazing Fire of the Heart." I made plans to go there on July 14 and come home on July

31. We would tell you about the surgery on August 1, two days before, as advised by the hospital's child psychologists. We hoped that your Dad would join us for at least a few days, but his work kept him in Boston.

The time we spent there is intrinsically tied to the surgery.

When we got the news about the surgery—it was like being spun into another space . . . we have been suspended in some kind of limbo. The first week or two afterwards was terrible. For a few days, I had the wrong statistics and thought that there was a 1 in 15 chance that you would not make it through the surgery. The grief was immense. Both your father and I did a great deal of crying. I feel very bad about the fact that you probably sensed a lot of this, even though you did not see or hear us cry. It must have worried you.

I was also worried about all the machines that would be hooked up to you in recovery. To operate, they will put you on a heart/lung bypass and stop your heart. When they are finished, you will be on a ventilator and unable to talk or cry. This particularly terrified me, as my mother was never able to get off the ventilator after her last surgery. You will also have drainage tubes, stomach tubes, pacer wires, and IVs.

We arrived at the ashram in time for the *Golden Tales* play. And after the play we were taken by one of the secretaries to the lower lobby to wait for our beloved Teacher. We were at one of the benches and She walked right over to you when She saw you. She reached Her hand out for you to take. When you did not take Her hand, She touched your head and asked, "Where's Dada?" Then She looked at me and walked away as She touched your hand again.

The next day was the beginning of Guru Purnima . . . there was a two-day saptah of *Om Namah Shivaya*. I longed to go to the *Guru Gita* that morning, as She was there, but did not. I spent as much time as you would in the saptah. On the last day of the saptah, She came into the temple to chant the *Shiva Arati* and we were there. That was nice . . . and then She went into the saptah— we went in the hall as well and you fell asleep for two and half hours! It was sometime during this time that Julia Carroll, a Reiki Master and friend initiated you into Reiki. She did this remotely from Houston, Texas. She is also doing distance healings on you during this time and plans to "be with you" during the surgery.

At the end of the saptah, She gave a formal darshan. As we stood in the darshan line, I began to sob . . . really deeply sob. You were so intent on seeing Her that you did not seem to notice. You ran ahead of me and waited at the front of the line—watching "Gummy" and waiting for me to get to the front of the line. I had stopped crying by the time I got there, and I was praying deeply and silently for fearlessness. I could hardly imagine how I would walk into the hospital with you and not have you feel my fear and anxiety. It seemed like an impossible thing to do. And yet, I knew that that is what I would have to do. I needed to get completely calm and centered about this in order to transmit that to you. I could not afford to be afraid.

After pranaming to Her and being bopped by Her peacock feathers, I started to move away, but you would not leave the chair. She laughed and said, "She doesn't want to leave. It's okay. Sit down there." She pointed to a space behind Swami V. We sat down, but you kept moving closer to Her and saying. "Excuse me, Gummy . . ." When She turned to you; you would have nothing to say! This happened a few times, and I tried to get you to sit down quietly. She looked at me and said, "It's okay, RELAX." And that became my mantra. After a few more interruptions, I told you that if you wanted to ask Gummy something you could tell Swamiji your question. You told him that you had a present for Gummy, but it was in your room. So Gummy asked a darshan attendant to drive us to Atma Nidhi to get Gemma's present!

You had collected a box of presents for Her. I bought a beautiful box with a heart on it and you filled it up. Your favorite shells. And from the toy store a red notepad with a kitty on it because Gummy writes notes sometimes. A pink ink pen. Some stickers. A red heart candle, because Gummy loves me. And your favorite—"Gummy Lobsters"!

You wrapped everything in wrapping paper that you made by painting paper . . . you wrapped it all with the pretty side in. Gummy and Swamiji unwrapped every single present right there . . . struggling through your love of scotch tape. And then Gummy gave you a great big teddy bear that you later named Gummy Bear.

She also called over Nivritti and asked me to "tell him everything."

We had a great stay. You went to Gokul children's house most mornings and loved it; and in the afternoons we played together. We went to the temple everyday.

One day I got very angry with you for talking in the temple and then climbing on top of me as I pranamed. I overreacted and had to apologize later. And we worked out a signal. If you were not able to be quiet in the temple, you would tap me on the shoulder and we would go. That pretty much worked. I had to acknowledge that I was very angry in general and had less patience with you than I should.

I met with Swami I. He said, of course you are angry with God that this is happening to your child!

I denied being angry with God. That was not acceptable to me. But that night, I realized that, yes, I was angry with God. I was sad and angry that your chest had to be cut open and that you would be in pain. As soon as I accepted this anger, it began to dissipate.

I also talked to him about trying to understand the lessons in this crisis. He reminded me to do lots of puja and pray for guidance. He also sent me to M.

M. is a great man. He is a quadriplegic that has lived in the ashram for many, many years. He has had two death experiences and spent a lot of time on ventilators and in hospitals.

M. was inspiring, to say the least. He reminded me that this was all in God's hands. He talked about how he loved his ventilator because it keeps him alive! He said that when you were having surgery you would be surrounded by angels and celestial beings . . . and that Gummy would be with you . . . he said it was Daddy and I that would need the help. He said you would probably be worried about us. When I told him that I was trying to see the doctor as God, but how was I actually going to turn you over to someone who would be cutting your chest open, he said, "Ah, you are still seeing the surgeon as separate!" What insight. I began to do puja to the surgeon and his team. "There's only one."

I was also reading everything I could get my hands on about heart surgery and especially open-heart surgery and children.

During the last darshan before going home, She asked me if I was staying in touch with Nivritti. Actually, I had not spoken to him after the first time; I thought there was not much to tell. And perhaps felt it unnecessary. She said somewhat sternly, but with love, "You have to learn to receive Grace, Shivani." Lot's of bopping.

As She left the hall, you wanted to go with Her, so K. scooped you up and took you to Her. She carried you for sometime as She walked behind the scenes and then before handing you back to K., Gummy kissed you and said, "Don't worry. You will be well." K. brought you back to me and told me about this.

Dad and I told you the first morning we woke up at home. We told you that your heart needed mending and that the doctors at the hospital needed to do surgery. We told you that we would be staying with you the whole time. You said, "Today?"

Later that same day, I took you to the hospital just to look around . . . we visited the playroom (where you saw children with tubes); we had lunch in the restaurant downstairs . . . we hung out in the lobby a bit . . . doing what the

Indians call "walking the turf." We just spent some time there and then left without any procedures or tests being done.

The next day we went back for Pre-op. We never saw the doctor because he was delayed in surgery. We were supposed to be the first case, 7 A.M. the next morning, but they called later and moved us to second case, 11:30 A.M., because we would then have a chance to meet the surgeon. Up to this point I had only spoken to him on the phone.

Maren, a recent friend from the Cape (mother of Alaina, another 3-year-old) met us at the hospital. She asked to come and it seemed a good idea to have someone that could help us if we needed it. We had to be there by 8 A.M. We all sat in the playroom trying to distract each other as much as possible. You asked Maren, "What are they going to do to me?" You had been so silent about it all with us. You had never asked us anything like this. I think you felt we might be withholding something . . . as we had been for weeks!

A nurse came for you and we went to a procedure room where they prepped you for an IV, and then we returned to the playroom to wait.

At about 11:30 A.M. the surgeon came in and asked if we had heard the bad news. He said the surgery had to be postponed because of lack of beds and nurses in the Cardiac Intensive Care. A dramatic shift.

As soon as this sank in and I could speak, I said, "Everything happens for the best." I knew immediately that the postponement was really because you were not in alignment with this yet.

When you heard it was postponed, you said, "What does that mean?"

Maren said "It means you can have some crackers, there is no surgery for you today."

You held up your wrist with the hospital ID bracelet on it and said: "Cut this off! I want crackers!"

Dr. Lillys met with Dad and I while you stayed with Maren in the playroom. He explained the surgery to us more completely and drew us a diagram. I had on a photo pin of an Indian saint and his eyes kept being drawn there.

Because we lived locally, we were put on a 24-hour notice to come in the first time Dr. Lillys had a cancellation. It was either that or reschedule for October.

We left the hospital and went straight to the meditation center . . . the center had chanted the *Guru Gita* that morning and was being kept open for devotees to come and pray or chant for you. We told them what had happened, we prayed for a few minutes ourselves, and then went to lunch with Maren.

By the time we got home, there was a message from the hospital that Dr.

Lillys had scheduled you for the following Friday, August 11. I called and asked if this would be first or second case, and she said it will be his only case—he scheduled you on his day off.

August 4
We've come down to North Falmouth for a few days. It is relaxing for all of us to be here.

August 5
Today, while sitting on the beach at Woodneck, I came across an article in the back of an old magazine about a little girl that had heart surgery. It was talking about a new technology that allowed for very small incisions for ASD repair. You also have a mitral valve repair, and so will need a larger incision, but the article was heaven sent. There were two pictures. One was of the little girl in the hospital before her surgery. She was wearing a hospital johnny; looking very worried and sad. Her mother was holding her . . . arms wrapped around her in a protective and nurturing way. The other photo was of the little girl running in a field, looking very happy. I showed you these photos and told you that the little girl had her heart fixed in the hospital. You said nothing, but never took your eyes off the pictures as I spoke about the feelings that the little girl might have. "She looks very sad to me. And maybe a little frightened. But, her mother is there with her holding her." etc. Then I pointed out the other photo. "This is the little girl a few weeks after her surgery. Look how happy she looks! Look at how she likes to run now! You'll be able to run like that after your heart is mended."

It was like a switch had been thrown. That evening, we went for a sunset walk and you were so playful and happy. The change was very dramatic and we realized just how anxious you had been.

August 12
Well, my dear one. You are in a very deep, morphine sleep. It is 3 A.M. Your dad took the first shift from 9 P.M. to 2 A.M., and now I am here with you until morning.

We arrived at the hospital at 6:15 A.M. yesterday. They took us down to pre-op holding at 7:15 A.M. Once there, the anesthesiologist came in and spoke to us. He was very nice, and wanted to listen to the Mantra that you would have on headphones during the surgery. Dr. Lillys had prepped everyone that this was important to us! He liked the Mantra very much, and asked where he could get it. Asked if he could go to Tower Records and look under "mantras"! We will leave this tape with him when we leave. His name is Dr. Barry Bussman and he is from South Africa.

He gave you a drug called versed . . . meant to relax you and cause you to forget the surgery. (I had mixed feelings about making you forget it, because I know on a deeper level, you cannot forget it.) You got very sleepy, very quickly. You were laughing . . . like you were drunk. I told you to watch for Gummy and you got a big smile on your face.

I gowned up and put on the blue surgical cap that looked like a blue shower cap. You thought that was very funny. You were laughing and slurring your words already, but tried to point to the cap and ask me "Why are you . . ." As soon as you were asleep, I picked you up and carried you into the Operating Room . . . along with two anesthesiologists and a nurse. I laid you on the operating table, and took your shirt off. They began to place stickers on to monitor you and gave you a mask with gas to really put you out.

After you were out, I kissed you, told you again to watch for Gummy, to watch for the light, told you that we loved you and would be right outside, and then I was escorted out of the OR. As I walked down the hall, I realized that I had the bunny in my hand that Gummy had given to you. I found Dad crying. It was hard for him to watch me walk away with you.

Then the wait began. I did the Mantra for a little while, and then began the *Guru Gita*. At 8:30 A.M. they came to tell us that they were doing the incision. At 9 A.M. they came to tell us that you were on the heart/lung bypass. We decided to go wait in the garden. It is a beautiful garden. I sat under a Redwood tree and finished the *Guru Gita*, while Dad did a japa walk around and around the garden.

While I was chanting, I forgot my intention to wrap you in light throughout the surgery—then I realized that I was wrapped in light. A white light surrounded me. All the prayers and grace were surrounding us all in light.

Just before 10 A.M. we went back up to the waiting area and they were just starting to look for us to tell us that your surgery was complete! You were off the heart bypass!

Soon, Dr. Lillys came out to talk to us while you were being closed up. He said it all went very well. He said it was one of the largest holes he had ever seen. Sixty percent of the septal wall between the atria was not there. Your heart has been working very, very hard just to keep you going! The mitral valve had ten stitches. There is still mild regurgitation at the mitral and tricuspid valves, but he expects the tricuspid to return to normal and there will only be a "whiff" of regurgitation at the mitral valve. The tricuspid valve had been pulled out of alignment because your heart was so oversized due to all the work it had to do.

We were able to see you at 11:30 A.M. We wrapped you in B.B.'s shawl. The Mantra was still playing through your headphones. You slept deeply until about 4 P.M.—then you began to flicker your eyes and move your toes and hands a bit, but it was 5:30 P.M. before you really woke up. You began to cry and look around at everything. You were very unhappy. Fortunately, the doctor was right there and checked to see if you could come off the ventilator. So you came off about half an hour after waking. At first we were told to leave the room while they took the ventilator tubes out. The nurse insisted that we leave. We started to go, but got only as far as the nurses station before realizing that we should not be leaving you alone for that. We went back to your bedside, but the nurse insisted that we would have to leave. I just said okay, we would wait for the doctor. When the doctor arrived, I told her we had to stay for this and she said we could stay. We had to step back away from you and the bed, but you knew we were there. What is the point of being there throughout the day if we have to leave when it gets tough for us?

Months later, I asked you what you remembered about the hospital and you recalled when "they" tried to make Daddy and me leave the room, and we wouldn't leave you.

You asked for water immediately and repeatedly. But the nurses would not let you have water for another four hours. They needed to be sure that you would not need to go back on the ventilator. Daddy held little water-soaked sponges to your mouth. Dad got you something to drink as soon as possible. You have been sleeping ever since. You have chosen to speak very little.

You woke again at about 4 A.M. I gave you a bit of water and asked you if you'd like to have the Mantra headphones back on. You shook your head no, but looked at me in a way that I knew there was something else. I said, "Do you want me to chant the Mantra to you?" You nodded, "yes." So I very softly chanted the Om Namah Shivaya in the Bupali Raga. It was just what we both needed. A wise little soul, you are.

Saturday

The next day is already a blur to me. (I am writing several weeks later now.) You received the last morphine at about 8 A.M.; slept most of the morning, and then on and off all afternoon. You pretty much remained silent. Perhaps a healing silence . . . perhaps just contemplative . . . trying to figure out what had happened to you. Mary Ann came by to see you. I got balloons from the gift shop from Auntie Elaine and Auntie Pat—a big blue dolphin and a beautiful huge butterfly—and hung them above your bed. You liked them a lot, but were still not really happy. We moved out of ICU and into a semiprivate room at about 5:30 P.M. The little girl in the room with you cried most of the night, and so you and I got very little sleep. Dad went home.

Sunday
Consequently, Sunday was not a great day—both you and I were very tired. And you had to have blood drawn and a set of x-rays taken.

We had a lot of visitors: Mary Ann came again, with two little stuffed monkeys. You were so miserable you did not even open the present while she was there. Maren, Al and Alaina came and we went to the garden with them; you in a big wagon, with the drainage apparatus rolling along beside you; and Aunt Elaine and Uncle Bob came to visit that evening.

A great nurse got you to walk to the door of your room and back Sunday evening . . . that was a big move, and you began to improve after that. It was hard to get you to walk at first; You did not want to do it.

You kept reaching out for me to pick you up and I had to keep backing away from you as you walked towards me holding up your arms. After the first trip to the door, you walked more easily. Dad got you up walking again an hour later.

Monday
Monday morning I got up and took a cup of tea into the playroom to read a bit. At 6:30, a little five-year-old boy came in with his mother, father and grandmother. He was about to have the same surgery. I was so moved. It was like being back in that time and space with you . . . entering the unknown. The father's eyes watered up when I spoke to him. I could feel their pain and anxiety. It is so hard to know your little one is going to be so vulnerable. So hard to hand your child over to someone you don't even know and let that person cut them open!

Monday morning they took out the drainage tubes. Gave you mor-phine again . . . you were very funny—bit like a drunken sailor . . . slurring your words just a bit and emphatically telling the nurse that you did not want any more needles, EVER.

You napped a bit, but played also. Your best friend Zoe came to visit with her Dad at about 6:30 to 8 P.M. And Jeanne came by that evening as well. Dr. Roxanne and Dr. Megan came for a long visit. Roxanne has spent so much time with us. She came both Saturday and Sunday, even though they were her days off. And tonight she sat with us for about an hour! She says you can go home tomorrow morning. This makes me a little bit nervous—it has all happened so quickly—I don't feel like I've gotten my feet on the hospital ground yet.

Tuesday

Packing! Dad arrived at 7 A.M. with bagels—waking us up! Eager to take you home! We were discharged at about 10 A.M. It was noon before we left. You wanted to play with the little girl in the next bed. Her name was Nicole. And then we all visited the little girl that had been next to you in ICU. You loved visiting other little girls. You gave Nicole the paper dolls that the child life specialist had made with you. You were so excited by them, and then turned around and gave them away! I was so proud of your open heartedness!

Then we were home! Alleluia! It was good to be there. You went immediately to your room and played there—very happy to be home. Later that day you danced around the living room.

Friday

All eager and full of gratitude, we went to the ashram. In our room we found a dozen pink roses for you and a huge teddy bear that is bigger than you are. Paul and I were in a state of overwhelm and both got very sick. We decided to go back home.

We were called into the Namaste Room that afternoon before we left. Paul and I were both sick and so we stood back about 8-10 feet away . . . Gemma went right to Gummy.

Gummy hugged her gently, asking both Gemma and I whether or not she still had pain. She kissed her several times. She said, "I love you. Did you know that I was remembering you during your surgery?"

Gemma gave Gummy a picture she'd painted for Her. Gummy was commenting on the colors and how beautiful it was, and Gemma said, "Turn it around. You are holding it upside down."

She picked Gemma up, saying. "Let's see if you have become lighter. Yes, you have become lighter." She asked to see the incision and Gemma let her lift her dress and see it. Gummy said it was beautiful. "You are looking very happy, Gemma. You are always very happy."

Then She told Gemma that she smelled like the Mantra. Once before

She told Gemma that she smelled like India. Gemma called me to come over to Gummy, too. She said, "They are standing back because they are ill."

I told Gurumayi that Gemma had the Mantra playing on headsets throughout the surgery. Paul added that we played the Darbari Raga and I corrected him—we played Darbari Raga only after she was conscious and in recovery—during the surgery we played the Bupali Raga. This correction made Her laugh.

Gummy hugged Gemma and kissed her many times—rubbing her back gently and then said that She would see her again soon. She wished us all a good trip and turned to go into Her house.

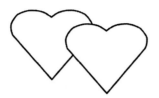

BREASTS
Kay

My practice almost always has a client suffering with cancer of the breast. This is a report about Kay. Kay was trained in advanced degrees of Reiki Touch Therapy, and she had breast cancer.

The phone rang as another friend and I were having afternoon tea and discussing various events of the day. I cheerfully answered the phone and at first thought no one was on the other end of the line. What I was interpreting as silence was a voice, a whisper, calling my name. It was Kay, a longtime friend. She had just come from her annual physical examination and her doctor found a lump in her breast. Kay's world took a sudden jolt as her life passed before her eyes. What had she done to cause this? Was there guilt? Had her diet not been proper? Did she not rest enough and have enjoyment of life? Her head immediately filled with these and many other questions.

Kay is an intelligent, practical and action-oriented individual. She quickly took charge and asked the doctor what was next. The doctor outlined many tests and informed Kay of her choices. After Kay left the doctor with as much information as possible, she called me. She was not her usual analytical, articulate self with me. After I took a couple of very deep breaths, internally calling upon my Guru to guide me, I asked her what was wrong. I pressed the phone receiver into my ear as she, robotlike, murmured the diagnosis. She had about three days for all the results of the tests to come in and during that time she wanted as much Reiki as could possibly be packed in. Of course. I asked her to come right over and stay as long as she wanted.

I set up the treatment table with comfortable sheepskins, lots of pillows and soft blankets. I was preparing for an infantlike setting. This is the vulnerability with a breast cancer diagnosis. I made sure my crystal scalpel was also available. Soothing music was playing on a low volume. I lit a scented candle and brought some fresh flowers in from the garden. Flower petals have a mission in addition to their beauty. This vital mission is to absorb negative energies. The phone was off the hook and the "In Session" sign was placed on the office door to ensure quiet and privacy. I had a teapot heating water for tea and selected some chamomile for calmness with a little added mint for vibrational lifting.

Kay arrived with a look on her face I will never forget. She was surrendering to whatever it took to get well. This was just an hour or so after hearing the announcement from her doctor. As previously stated, Kay is intelligent, astute and action oriented. We shared a cup of tea as she related the afternoon's events. She mostly stared at the floor or the wall because eye contact with me would make it more real. After about a half hour of discussion I invited her onto the Reiki table.

A Reiki Touch Therapy session always begins with the head. Mental thought forms create the physical imbalance. We create our own reality as much as we would like to think otherwise. I placed my hands on Kay's head and checked out the energy patterns in her body. They were even except around the designated breast. I found myself wishing that I was still practicing the psychic surgery so I could just open her body and go get this lump, this threatening tumor. Instead I did a half hour or so of Reiki on the breast. Reiki brings balance and harmony to the body, mind and soul. Reiki addresses the source of imbalances. So, many things occur as the treatment is administered.

After I felt the breast area was full of Reiki energy, I told Kay that I was going to do etheric surgery on the lump. She was adamant that anything I could do would be welcome. I held my crystal scalpel in my hands and offered my work to my Guru, to God and to the ascended Tibetan Reiki Masters. I prayed for skill, guidance and dharma, or right action.

The etheric body is the invisible body just outside the physical body. It contains virtually all components of the physical body except for the density and physicality of it. Generally, the lump or tumor will appear in the etheric three to six months before manifesting in physical form. So, this tumor had been in Kay's etheric space just waiting for an opportunity to enter her physical body.

When I felt the energies of all invited were aligned I deftly pointed the crystal at the newly discovered lump in Kay's breast. I began at the outermost point and worked in toward the tumor. With great focus, praying constantly, I began to separate the energetic portion of the tumor that had attached itself to the outer areas of the breast. You might imagine a stone thrown into a pond creating concentric circles around where it entered the water. The outer circles are affected energetically, but not physically, by the object in question. I addressed these adjoining areas by gently but thoroughly cutting and separating the tumor from the rest of the breast. I must isolate the tumor in order to lift it out. As I slowly cut around the periphery, I moved closer and closer into the tumor area. Finally, the tumor was isolated and free of all connections to the other tissues.

I put a white light in the area and then wrapped what I call a Reiki bandage around the tumor itself. The Reiki bandage is actually made of ectoplasm, which contains all the components of life force. It is usually whitish in color, but as I add Reiki to it, it becomes a beautiful emerald green. The bandage varies in thickness and in width based on the size and seriousness of the disease or injury. This bandage was thin, about a half-inch wide, but also about a half-inch thick, and I wrapped it around several times. The reason for multiple layers is that a diseased tissue will rapidly absorb the Reiki bandage in an attempt to heal and make itself whole.

The tumor was now separated from the breast and bandaged all around. I put the scalpel aside and with my fingers gently lifted it out and put it aside onto a silver plate. I would later bury it. Yes, it is invisible and etheric, and it also exists. At the burial it would be thanked for the message Kay needed to alter her life. I would assure the tumor that it had done its job, that it need not return and that it could now rest in peace.

Kay, being emotionally exhausted, had fallen asleep during this process. She very much wanted to stay awake and observe but could not. She now stirred, opened her eyes and inquired as to the stage of the process. I quietly told her it was over, that the etheric tumor was now out of her body. We both hoped that now the surgery would not be necessary. Sometimes it is not, but this time it was. The tumor was large. There was a history of breast cancer in her family and everyone felt that all avenues should be explored. This is individual choice and I always support that.

During her surgery another Reiki Master was granted some space in the hospital operating room to perform distant energy focusing Reiki during the surgical process. We were all very pleased with that. The surgery went much quicker and smoother than the doctors had predicted, as did her rapid recovery. We felt the Reiki had successfully done its part.

Kay decided to continue with a short chemotherapy and radiation regime.

She never missed a day of work, had normal energy and her attitude about her future was positive and never wavered. She took a couple of extended trips with friends and kept up with strenuous tourist-type endeavors.

Kay radically changed her life. She changed her career, her home location, and even her boyfriend. She is now comfortably established in her new life, wisely having regular mammograms and checkups. She is very happy and serene and accepts life with more peace and calmness than before this event.

Dr. Carl Simonton, an oncologist and cancer visualization therapist, states in his books and lectures several important changes one must make.

He says to radically change your life. Stop what you have been doing and begin something radically new. He also says to thoroughly enjoy everything you do, before you do it, while you are doing it and after you have finished it. If any part of this is not enjoyable then do not do it.

He further states not to do anything you do not want to do. This last one involves an attitude change because life sometimes presents itself with something unavoidable. Then, adopt the "this too, shall pass" attitude.

Cancer - A Gift?

My phone rings with death and dying calls. Years ago, physicians and friends queried this, wondering why my calls did not concern common headaches or sprained ankles. This I attribute to karma; karma with the individuals and karma with the imbalances. Well over ninety percent of my clients have a terminal diagnosis of cancer. Over the years, observing the individuals' spiritual growth during the healing process, the clients evolve into a space of truth, a oneness with God, a sense of contentment and peace. Fear dissolves into trusting the process. The gift of life, with its precious and multifaceted moments, brings a greater awareness within and without.

I have come to assess this as a gift. If one suddenly loses their life-breath in an automobile accident or a heart attack, there has been no "real time" conscious opportunity to explore or to correct any aspect of this life. When someone is diagnosed with cancer, all the denial, anger, grief, acceptance and other processes are addressed. In my experience this is an invaluable gift; the gift of time to assess, correct and make amends prior to leaving the body. Once I asked a cancer client what her relationship was to God. She was embarrassed by the question and defiantly stated that she was a Methodist. A few weeks later, arriving for her appointments with the red radiation marks and ill from chemotherapy, she humbly asked me how to establish a relationship to God. When one is faced with a mortality issue, whether they invite it or not, they definitely want to know what is next and appreciate any information you, as a healer and counselor, can offer.

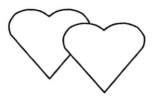

PANCREAS
Kenneth

At age forty-one Kenneth had already had one bout with cancer. He was an angry and fearful man who stuffed all this inside. Outside he was gentle, kind and had great wisdom. All his life he had been in competition for his father's attention. According to Ken, and by all appearances, his father liked his brother best.

Because of thyroid cancer eight years before, he was very mindful of his diet. He loved food and truly missed the rich sauces and most of all, ice cream. His wife was very diligent in preparing organic and natural meals for him. They were both psychologists and worked with special education children in school. Kenneth had decided, against his wife's wishes, that there would be no children of their own.

He telephoned one day and I had a cancellation, so told him to come right over. He did not say what the appointment was for. I stood at the office window and watched as he parked his car. He seemed a little cautious about his body and his gait was off balance. Then I saw his face. It was gray. I then observed his torso and noted that one side was distended. I sighed deeply, and felt an inner sob touch my heart.

A big, wide smile covered his face as he saw me. I could sense that his body was heaving a sigh of relief. Finally, someone who knew his pain and supported him with his physical and emotional plight. I returned his smile. We were happy to see each other, but we were also smiling to keep from crying.

I gave him a cup of chamomile tea, which he always requested and expected. He sat on the sofa and I sat across the room, both secure within the pink painted walls. The warm rays of the sun were shining in over the white louvered blinds. He sat in silence for quite a while, just sipping his tea. I was glad. It was a comfortable quiet space and it gave me some time to assess his energy and body language. After a bit, he took a long and deep breath and said, "I have pancreatic cancer."

Another inner sob leapt from my heart. Thank goodness I kept the professional poker face. Being a psychologist and a caretaker himself, he would have felt guilty for making me feel sad and the tables would have turned. I remained quiet and waited for him to go on.

He said his father had finally caught up with him but he was going to have the last laugh. He was going to die before his father, and his father would have to live with the guilt of favoring his brother. Kenneth was both jubilent and bitter about this.

Kenneth and I had known each other for eight years, and he had survived cancer before. I asked him what he wanted from me; "hearts and flowers" or "nuts and bolts." He replied, "Nuts and bolts." I asked him what preference he had about his death projections. He bitterly answered that he would love to just be mowing the yard in the hot sun and have a heart attack, quick and easy. But he said that that would not be the way it was. He would not have quick and easy, he would have a long, slow and painful death. I felt he had written his script.

We talked about having his affairs in order, insurance, a will, final resting plans; practical matters. We discussed the information his wife had. Not much. I asked him if he wanted her to be trained in Reiki Touch Therapy so she could assist him in maintaining his energy between his appointments. He thought that was a good idea.

The next visit Ken brought his wife, Mary, in for training. She did not know he had pancreatic cancer and I let him talk me into telling her. She was very quiet; showing emotion was not something she did. After the training she left and Kenneth stayed for his Reiki treatment.

Kenneth, in my opinion, gave himself this cancer. There are a lot of ways to consider this, but this was my experience. He told me he had been to one hospital for surgery, but nothing was found. He was quite angry with the doctors because he knew it was a mistake; that they just couldn't find it.

He was confident that I would find it and then he could go back to the doctors and give them more information so they could operate again. My hands definitely found an imbalance. Kenneth was certainly in pain. I focused on the area where my hands responded the most. I could also "see" inside his body. The pancreas was almost closed together on either end and the ducts were closed due to swelling and inflammation. The liver and spleen also seemed in jeopardy.

I used my crystal scalpel and a couple of other crystals that had rounded and polished edges. Slowly I inserted the crystal scalpel into one end of the pancreas and gently forced it open to allow the fluids to move in and out. I inserted the other crystal into this opening to gently provide a stretch so the opening would remain so. I repeated this process at the other end of the pancreas. In etheric surgery, even though the crystals are dense, tangible instruments in my hands, inside his body they would conform and obey any instructions given to them. One of the attributes of crystals is that they can be programmed. I did Reiki after this procedure and that also reduced the swelling and helped with the pain. After the treatment I left the two inner crystals in place to provide openings for the flow from connecting organs.

Kenneth came every day for the twenty-one-day cancer treatment plan. His color was better, his distention was less and his attitude was better. I noticed this and wondered if he did. After all, he did not want to be well or to be happy. He had far too much vested in dying this painful death. He just wanted to convince the doctors that he had cancer and in a paradoxical way wanted to take his wife on a trip to Africa! He felt that he owed her that much since he refused to have any children.

After the twenty-one days, Kenneth entered a different hospital and convinced them to operate. They found absolutely nothing except one slightly swollen lymph node that could be treated with antibiotics. He was pretty angry with me. He said that he did not want me to make him well, but just to give the doctors some information to prove he had this cancer.

I suggested that he take this opportunity, while he was "in remission" to take Mary on the long-awaited trip to Africa. He thought that was a great idea as he was not currently in pain and had some energy for a vacation.

About two weeks later I had a call from Mary. Kenneth had experienced major pain on the trip. They had not even reached Africa, just Europe, but immediately returned because his cancer had come back. I asked her which hospital he was in and went there right away. They were just wheeling him back to his room after a long surgery. He had an incision stretching almost the length of his torso. Mary informed me that he was full of cancer and that it was inoperable. This was his third surgery and the first time anyone had found anything and now it was inoperable. He was winning.

As Kenneth stirred and turned to see me by his bed I could quickly discern that he had very mixed feelings. His wife was positive that he would want me there to give him Reiki treatments. He was caught. What to do? His surgeon and another doctor came in and observed me doing the Reiki on Kenneth. Kenneth very proudly introduced me as his Reiki Master and explained to these doctors just what Reiki was. The doctors were appropriately interested and kind and said they were glad to meet me.

Kenneth was happy. He had his legitimate cancer. It was inoperable and he was going to die. That would show his father!

Kenneth was in the hospital for three weeks. I was coming up there every day. He was getting better and the doctors and nurses found that very interesting. Kenneth realized it, too. And even though he liked my company, he did not want to get well.

On my next visit he angrily told me to never see him again, ever. We were the only ones in the room. He would not meet my eyes. He was determined and had made up his mind. No more Julia and no more Reiki.

Mary was not informed of this decision and was perplexed as to why I was not coming to the hospital. Kenneth could not tell her that he did not want to live and be with her as her husband. Kenneth and I had client confidentiality, so I could not tell Mary either. It was very difficult. Mary became angry with me and I was stuck with professional confidentiality.

Kenneth was taken home to die. He had, as he predicted, his long, slow, painful death experience. He had a feeding tube putting food in for twelve hours and then another tube to take it out. He was in and out of a comatose state for another three weeks or so. Mary would leave messages on my phone informing me of how bad he was and how much he needed me to come and treat him. I never returned the phone calls.

To this day, almost twenty years later, I have tortured myself over the decision not to tell her that her husband told me he never wanted to see me again. So, Mary, if you ever read this, please know that I felt I had to honor Kenneth's last wishes. Thank you.

Kenneth left me his journal. In it he described his painful growing up with a wealthy father who favored his brother. Kenneth often spoke of wanting his father to give him a very large sum of money so Kenneth could feel his love and approval. Then, in Kenneth's understanding, this would give him more self-respect. Kenneth said that his mother programmed him to be sickly and in order for him to get attention he had to be sick.

I cannot begin to tell you the number of children, of all ages, who have died, one way or the other, because of feeling unloved by their parents. Children have been terminally ill, have taken their lives or have been institutionalized from psychological disorders, all due to parental arguments, emotional abuse or neglect. I have been part of many family situations where the child had to side with one or the other parent. Children are like sponges and absorb the good and the bad of the parent role. Parents incorrectly think that their words, sometimes at high decibels, have no effect on the child in the home. Children cannot take mixed messages from parents. Children are not little adults; they are children who must have reasonable enjoyment, security and the love of a primary caregiver in order to mature and thrive.

LUNGS
Dylan

Thithis chapter will be in the form of a diary. In some places it may not seem to have a continuous flow. This client survived, with the will of a strong soldier, and the stature of a young prince, for about two years. I selected segments that seemed to capture his essence, his circumstances, his beauty and love of life, and ultimately his death. Dylan was in his early twenties when he became my client. We worked together for his wellness program virtually every day.

A select group of Reiki Masters and Reiki Professional Degrees teamed together to provide a twenty-four-hour energy system for him. Softly and sweetly I invite you to enter Dylan's last few months on this good ship Earth. Be with him as he struggled. Join his amazing insight and acceptance at the end. Note the communication exchange both before and after his passing. This is a reverent chapter, designed to honor his memory with dignity. With respect to him, I offer this to you.

"Dylan, where are you this evening? I wonder if you are sensing a big construction project going on in your body. I suspect you are since it was your idea in the first place. Yes?"

The body is a complex mechanism. What is important for me is the consciousness of each component . . . the cell, the mitochondria in the cell, which gives the cell energy, the respiratory chain, the type I neumocyte, many things. And, in my experience, communication can be established to find precisely what and how to utilize them in his body to optimize his wellness process.

So, that is what I will do now. I will go and bring him to me and present this information to him—to his mind, to his body and to his spirit. Then I will break that down to smaller parts and go to the etheric grid that is set up and investigate how this information can be used in the lungs.

One of the mysteries of the mitochondria is that their enzymes catalyze the citric acid cycle of reactions which provide about 95 percent of the cell's energy supply. This greatly enhances and augments the cell's capability to do the job it is designed to do.

In addition, the mitochondria design supports the principle that organization is a foundation stone and a vital characteristic of life.

The more I read the more I discover about this marvelous, mighty mitochondria. I have a belief system that if we endow anything with power and a purpose then it is infused with such and functions accordingly. I am doing this with the mitochondria. As I instruct them to form a fence around your lungs and various situations in your lungs, they already have an innate direction. I add a spiritual element to their direction by endowing them with higher powers. I decided to initiate the masses of mitochondria in your lungs so they will have a connection to the highly refined healing energy of Reiki. This combines with what their purpose is anyway. In searching for all avenues of modalities I turned a page that illustrated the various pleura. Since the pleura are inside this particular grid, I thought the mitochondria also should be there. There are visceral pleura covering your lungs, parietal pleura lining the walls of your chest cavity, and the pleural space between the visceral and the parietal. That is a lot of space and some of it has been previously addressed in your health process, so I thought we should cover our bases and attend to those, also . . . okay?

I thanked the mitochondria for the work it did last night in surrounding the lungs individually and together, and literally covering the splotchy patches, mostly in the left lung. I praised them for their work and told them to stay positioned until I told them otherwise. They are very dutiful, very matter of fact and know their job.

Then I called in a whole new etheric troop for the pleura, placed them in the proper arenas, asked them to fence off the respective territories, and to do what they were created to do. Again, they were very orderly and obedient and also happy to be there for a specific duty. They felt proud to serve!

I then just placed my hands on your lungs, back and front, and gave you Reiki. I tell you, my hands were just vibrating and pulsating with new energy. I could both sense and feel movement going on. Pretty great.

I will be cautious about the 21-breath process while we concentrate on the mitochondria stage. You can let me know if you need it . . . and we will do it slowly and carefully.

I did not communicate with him in the same manner tonight as I had been. It was more at a distance, as an observer.

There are a lot of things going on in his body all at once. Before he left for the hospital there was a shift, mentally and emotionally, which would affect the rest of the body, too. This had to happen because changes were happening . . . new experiences were being introduced. He has a high intelligence, a questioning mind and these happenings had to be thought out almost while they were happening. So an overlap of thought and action.

We, the Reiki Masters, and the patient, and the family and the doctors knew this would be a "heavy" treatment. The Reiki Masters thought he would be sick from this—nausea, dizziness, disorientation, and low energy. We worked so he would not be so sick . . . for a lot of reasons . . . to be well enough to go through the treatments, to travel back and forth for the treatments, and to have a backlog of energy to continue his wellness process with the new medication.

He, himself, has created this new Reiki with the grids and the mitochondria. Very detailed, very complete, very thorough. And, at the same time has wanted "bedtime stories" and sweet songs. There is a tenderness that anyone who is going through this great battle would have . . . a vulnerability that allows strength and beauty through the pain.

I really see the depression as an outreach of the tiredness and the rethinking of his wellness process. Plus, remember the anniversary is coming up. That is a very real impactful happening. This is a primary focus for me right now to ease him, body, mind and spirit into, through and past the onset of this experience. My intent, along with the mitochondria grid process is to hold him in a space of healing, love and protection in every way possible during this anniversary period. Most important. It is almost as if I am holding my breath and sneaking him past a critical memory zone.

At the same time, we all are acutely aware of his needs and as healers, are diligently serving him with what we know how to do . . . Reiki.

That is what I will do more of now . . . goodnight.

Hi,

I spoke to your mom tonight. She is so loving and sweet, and worried and concerned. A true mom, don't you think? She asked me some valid questions as to the sequence of the healings. I told her that they had recently changed somewhat due to the process of the mitochondria and its workings. What I am doing is getting intuitive messages from you during the day, regarding what is going on with you and if you have something specific for me to address. With that information I have been doing some research so I will have answers for you and for me, as to how and what to do with this new "landscape," as your mom calls it.

Then I bring this written information home, do protection on myself, then on you, and go into meditation. The written information then begins to reveal itself to me visually, in pictures. I ask the pictures questions so I can be clear as to the direction and the interpretation of the written information. Sometimes I am interrupted and write it down while I still have you in my space. Sometimes I close you up in my hands and write what I have experienced . . . then, I go back and get you again. Recently, there has been a lot of traveling . . . sometimes several times during the night. This particular "landscape" is powerful and exacting and I want to make sure I am covering all the bases. You seem to know what needs to be done and I am following your directions in many ways. I do believe that your angels also are guiding you and maybe they are guiding me, too.

Ah, ha! Remember when I asked his angels if I could be a mediator for them and they could tell me what to do? This is astounding! I do believe that the mitochondria process began after I asked them for help! Amazing!

I recall telling you the other day, that I had been noticing the mitochondria changing shapes, going from elongated to fat and squatty looking. Today, in the book on cells I read that they change shape constantly. It just has to do with the inner process in the mitochondria. No particular reason that I saw today, except that there are no accidents.

In addition to the mitochondria I read that there is an epithelial cell that serves as a barrier function in the lining of the lung. This cell is called a "type I neumocyte" and it lines the air space of the lungs. I will do meditation on this to see if this information is supposed to combine with the mitochondrion functions.

Another sentence that leapt out from the Cell book was: "The enzymes of the respiratory chain are in the inner mitochondrial cristae, essential to the oxidative phosphoralation, which generates a higher percentage of ATP." ATP is adenosine triphosphate and it contains three phosphate groups. Two of these are high-energy bonds, which release active energy to perform cellular work, actually giving energy to the cells.

I think, overall, if we can make the healing process accelerate, then the depression will subside. I really do not think it can work the other way around right now.

When I contacted him I expected to get in on a microlevel, especially since I had been reading and thinking about that.

However, I immediately went to the top of his head. It was hot and I saw a reddish lining under his scalp. It seemed that there was a fever and that his temperature was a bit escalated. I asked his body why. Then I was shown the carotid arteries and jugular veins inside his neck, leading to his head. They were sluggish. I asked what was going on. They said that there was not enough oxygen getting to his blood going to and from his head. So, he would be slowed down in his thinking and acting processes. I asked if there was any dis-ease in the head and was told no . . . that it was an oxygen situation.

I asked for guidance and placed both my hands on the front of his lungs. I raised and lowered my hands in sync with his breathing. I put my hands on the back of his lungs and did the same . . . then on the sides, under his armpits and did the same. I also did an acupressure point technique inside his armpit. That is massaging clockwise three times and then massaging counter-clockwise three times and holding it for a count of 30 seconds. Then, go to the other arm. This increases the blood flow both to and from the heart to the arteries and veins. Since it is an upper body technique then the upper body is affected. The blood began to flow properly right away and his head cooled off.

Wondering what was next—since this was a surprise—I just put my hands on his lungs again. A soft pink energy radiated from my hands into his lungs and also surrounding his lungs. I then noticed the grid and that it was filling up with the pink energy. It conveyed to me that this pink energy is a love energy and that is what makes the cells have the consciousness to communi-cate with each other. Okay.

I then filled his whole body with pink energy followed by Reiki green energy. I allowed this combination of colored energy to expand outside his body, to provide an abundance of both loving pink and healing green energy.

I waited to see if I would get further instructions. I asked the mitochondria if I should do something. They said they knew what to do and were just fine. I moved toward the type I neumocytes for the lining of the air space of the lungs and was told not to do that now, that tonight only the basics were needed, and that was done, just to keep the protection sealed, the acupressure points activated and the pink and green energy available.

So, it was a very different scene than I was expecting. We will see what tomorrow brings.

Have you noticed any slower speech process or foggy thinking? Let me know if you notice this. The acupressure points are excellent for increasing the blood flow.

When I had you in my hands I talked to you about all the things I just mentioned. They are for you to contemplate.

I first checked to see how the supply of pink love energy and the green healing energy was. It needed a little replenishing so I did that. There was plenty inside but I added some outside your precious body.

Then I checked on your oxygen process and your blood situation with the oxygen. I did the acupressure points again as I did last night. I had been doing them periodically during the day also. I looked inside your arteries and veins leading from your heart to your head. Then I blew bubbles inside the arteries to aerate the blood, which increases the oxygen in the blood. I put my hands on the sides of your neck to warm up the vessels so the blood would flow faster and easier. Then I did Reiki on your head. It was not red or hot tonight.

I put my hands on your heart and did Reiki on it for a while and encouraged it to pump the blood at the rate it should be for your healing process. Then I traced my hands from the heart over the main arteries and veins that lead from the heart, first to the upper body, then to the lower body. I also blew air into the vessels at the heart so they would all be aerated as they circulate through your body.

The grids were checked and the mitochondria were checked. All were very intact and very busy. There are a couple of layers on the splotchy patches that will be ready to scrub off in a day or so . . . but not tonight. They have to be handled with care.

Well, my sweet, you are taking the energy exactly where you need it. I fully expect your platelets to be just fine. What about your hemoglobin? Is it being checked? It should also be fine. Let me know . . . okay? I really wish that I could actually see you and hold you. I also realize that those who are right with you feel the same way. Fear can produce separation and love can dissolve that separation. Consider accepting all the love that people can give to you. It will have a wonderful impact on your well-being. Stress connected to any illness can constrict body, mind and spirit functions. Again, love can dissolve that stress.

You were created in love, you are loved now and you have that love in you. Will you put yourself into this love and this loving state? You can still have your anger at your illness. That anger is justified. You can be totally pissed at this turn of events in your young life. That is honest and that is your truth. And, the love must be the stronger point.

I would also like for you to ask your body what it needs from you to be your friend. And, I would like your body to ask you what you need from it to be your body's friend. Then, you can ask life what it wants from you and you can tell life what you want from it. That will move toward establishing peace and equanimity in your body, mind and soul.

The grid is set . . . the mitochondria are eagerly and enthusiastically doing their work. All the other scientific elements are active and aware.

Think about your vision, your dream for your life. Forgive yourself for this illness, forgive yourself for the anger, forgive yourself for what you define as time that is lost. There is nothing you can change about what is . . . but you can take a deep breath, accept where you are and go forward in a different way . . . a way of love.

So, another process, which will lead to another process, which could lead to another process. You are up to it. Do not worry. You are strong. It is indicative of the anniversary month that some things may remind you of that first occurrence. Think long term.

I personally wish you were not having a general anesthesia for the catheter. Generals are hard on the lungs. That is something we will overcome. It may seem like a setback, because you are recovering from the treatment and this is almost like an overlap of processes before you fully bounce back. It is necessary though, so, bear up. As I said, you are up to it. Just have patience.

I believe in a positive, optimistic, healing approach and I work in that frame. In that light, I want to share with you a message that I have been intuitively receiving for about two weeks. There are still things to go through. But, the message that I am getting is that you will be in complete remission by December. You will earn this . . . it will not be easy from now until then . . . but the reward will be there. Keep that goal in mind. And, other than your Mom knowing it, I think it best to hold that energy information to yourself.

Tonight I placed my hands on your lungs with the intent of filling them completely full of Reiki to prepare you for the general anesthetic. I filled each part of the grid with Reiki green healing energy in addition to the pink loving energy already in place. I instructed the mitochondria to be alert and active for the onslaught of yet another invasion of your sweet body. I asked them to be in abundant numbers and to form a protective blanket over your lungs and inside your lungs. I asked them to be prepared to please work overtime so this anesthetic energy will not slow you down.

I also did the acupressure points and aerated your blood so you will have more energy. It will seem as if you have precious little energy, Dylan, but remember you are truly very strong and have lots of reserve. I will set up an energy field to fill you all night long to get you ready for tomorrow.

You have been giving me a song . . . "Night and day, deep in the heart of me," then that phrase repeats . . . and there is humming. I don't know the other words. You have been giving that to me for about three to four nights.

So, I will be in touch with you tomorrow . . . goodnight, my prince.

I had a message from another Reiki Master mentioning some water in your lungs. I checked on that tonight and it is the moisture I have always seen the little beings fan with their wings to keep it dry. Now, it is possible that some fluid is collecting in your pleura, but I am sure the doctors are on top of that. We all work together, you know.

It felt as if your blood was flowing quicker and more smoothly throughout the whole circulatory system tonight. And, I still gently traced the circulatory route from your heart to all the major arteries and veins. I also did the under arm acupressure points which increases circulation anyway. I blew gently on your heart and held my hands there for a long time. I was kind of giving you oxygen by osmosis.

The grid is still moving on its own and seems to be molding to your form. I filled each grid with loving pink heart energy and also the Reiki green energy. The mitochondria are still gathering and moving closer to each other in a blanketlike fashion inside and outside your lungs. They are on a mission, you know.

I did the 21-breath process. All the breaths were basically short, but that is okay. Sometimes the body knows what to conserve and what to use. I also reinforced your protection spheres and filled them with Reiki green energy. I blew the energy into each sphere to provide another way for you to receive oxygen. Goodnight, my precious prince, may you have sweet dreams. Think long term . . .

I have been building up a shield, which has open spaces in it for the radiation. This shield is green, of course, and has more than one thickness. The layers shift just slightly to lessen the direct onslaught of the radiation. The Reiki will monitor the volume control and will alter the layers that will soften the radiation impact.

The Reiki layers are also cool, which is important because frequently radiation can be hot, sometimes causing a sunburn-type effect. I feel your body is vulnerable and would rather not have anything severe just now. I pray that even though the oxygen is a bother that your breathing has evened out . . . and you have relaxed to depend on it rather than you doing it all. I do know that with activity it has to settle again, but overall I feel it is easier on you.

Yes, I will convey a message. "It is everyone's responsibility, even mine. I am human and so is everyone here . . . the truth is shared." All right, anything else. "Tell them to be gentle with themselves." Okay.

See you later . . . my friend.

Thank you for the dream last night.

Today I saw you in the hospital receiving blood. I asked you how you were. You said that you were cold. I asked where you were cold. You said all over. I asked you if you had asked anyone for a blanket. You said, yes, but it had not helped. I told you that the Reiki would warm you and I would do that for you. You said, "good." Later, you said it helped a little, but not completely.

I asked you what else was going on. You said your stomach was bothering you . . . like a knot in your stomach . . . then pain. I asked if you knew what was causing it. You said "no." I asked you about your leg. You said it was cold, too. I rubbed it gently, which warmed it up, and you said, "You can't do that all the time." I answered, "Not all the time, but a lot."

I sent the energy in through the top of his head for the inside of his body, then outside for the outside of his body. Then, put him inside my hands for the energy to merge. He seemed to rest. Still anxiety, difficult breathing, agitation . . . I did the 21-breath process again, very slowly. When it was time to close I asked him if he wanted to stay in my hands or not . . . he said that he did want to. I felt him all the way up to the mid-forearm on my right hand, less on the left hand.

Sometime during the night the dream returned. Again my bed was right by his. I did have a different tee shirt on, which he noticed. I sat on the side of my bed, facing his bed. He was resting with his eyes open. I looked at him. He said, "What?"

I said, "That is a good word, let's turn it around."

"Okay," he said, "I like games."

So, I said, "What is going on, really going on, truly going on?"

"Truly going on?" he sounded sarcastic. "There is no truth in this house! This is why I am sick, and angry; I am sick and angry that I am truth and no one is listening. Everyone is dead here and I am the only one acting like it . . . but everyone is dead."

"What do you mean, Dylan, that everyone is dead?"

"Everyone is dead to the truth, there is no truth here and it is killing me. I think it is killing them, too, but mostly me."

I said, "Everyone's truth is different, Dylan."

"Everyone's path in life is different." He said, "But I came here to show them and they won't listen, they are not paying attention, even now."

I said, "Tell me what you want them to listen to, perhaps I can share it in some way."

"They won't listen to you if they won't listen to me."

"Try, just tell me, please."

"It is so simple, they just need to listen to truth, that's all."

"Can you say it another way, Dylan, this may be too simple?"

"No, that's all."

Then, the dream switched to another scene. I saw Dylan on a train going across water on a red bridge . . . like the San Francisco Bridge. He was going to a hotel for a party or an event. The train was about to pass the station where he would get off, but it was going the opposite direction. He made the train stop anyway and got off. Then he realized he was stuck when he saw no other trains in sight. Several cars passed and strongly encouraged him to get in; he would not. One car, driven by a very large, black lady with three screaming children, stopped and demanded that he get in, that it was the only way he could get to the hotel, that no other train was coming. Dylan could not believe his eyes . . . that he had to get into that car with those loud children. But, the lady hopped out of her car, opened the back door and he got in. He had to hold a two-year-old, give her a bottle and calm her down. He was amazed at how adeptly he did that and was quite pleased with himself. The other two children crowded around him. He liked that, too.

When they reached the hotel, suddenly I was there again. He stood in front of me and looked at me a long time. He asked if I would stay with him the whole way. Our eyes were deeply intense. I said, "I always do, and, yes, I will, as long as you want or need me."

He smiled.

Dear Lilly,

I wish you well today. I wish you comfort, serenity, centeredness and balance. I wish for you a strong heart, a strong back, a strong voice, to be in the presence of love, to be protected from outside sources, to be firm, yet flexible. I give to you today, my friend, the mother of Dylan, healing energy in the form of Reiki Touch Therapy.

As you stand before me, facing me, I wrap you in a healing, energized shawl of translucent, glimmering and pulsating Reiki. I wrap your head, your lovely hair, and gentle face . . . only your eyes show. Eyes that see, perceive and understand. Calm eyes, frightened eyes, prepared and unprepared, open and closed eyes. There is an awareness of your heart, in pain, and your breasts that no longer give milk. The Reiki knows, envelopes, heals and supplies your needs. The wrapping is like that of fine, gold threaded silk, gentle around your stomach and torso, and gracefully falling around your legs and princess feet.

You look radiant, secure that you are lovingly wrapped and in a state of healing.

Be well . . . be comforted . . . be safe . . . be secure . . . be loved.

Hey, guy,

So, your world is topsy-turvy. You are absolutely beside yourself with "what to do?" Grasping at straws . . . do this? Do that? So much already done and for what? You are furious and sad, frustrated and confused, and you are not going to not do anything that is offered to you. So the new medication, samarium radioisotope, and stem cells . . . well, why not?

You feel like hitting things, throwing things, being absolutely out of control. All of this can be done . . . go ahead . . . why not? Do whatever you feel like doing, it is what you need to do right now.

You will feel, in some way, that you are "just going through the motions," getting the new treatment. You will doubt it, doubt yourself, doubt everyone and everything around you. You have to do that, too. You have to do whatever comes to you that you think expresses who you are and what you have to do now. Others around you are experiencing similar reactions so you will be understood.

The Reiki Master team has wrapped your room and your whole house in the Reiki green energy bandage. We have walked through the house energizing. We ask and give blessings to all within. We ask and give blessings for you, your new treatment, and for your courage and commitment to your healing process. We ask the sun to shine brightly on you and your home for warm energy . . . we ask the moon to shine its moonbeams at night to calm the energy in the house for everyone.

Play music, have flowers, open the curtains, invite life in.

See you later, my friend.

Dearest Lilly,

I held you today between my hands supporting you with Reiki energy. Just before dawn I became a pedestal and your feet stood on my hands. You were held high as I turned so the rising sun would light up your face as the first rays beamed over the horizon. The warm sunlight approached you, embraced you, penetrated and permeated your body, mind and spirit. You stood so strong, being blessed by the shining light on your beingness. At sunset you bowed in reverence to the light that is, was and will always be and offered gratitude.

Even before the sun set the moon was allowing you a preview of the night light, so magical. The moon crept silently over the treetops. You stood very firmly, anticipating, watching, waiting for the fullness that was approaching. Soon the moon owned the skies and everything, even the stars, reflected this moonlight. You stood; open, in wonder and in awe at the mystical moon. I do not know who captured each other's attention first, but all of a sudden, you and the moon were merging. The moon was so milky, with the nectar of life, and you dove in. You swam so freely, with abandon . . . all the strokes, diving deeply, not needing to breathe, like a fish.

The moon filled you with its essence and you were replenished. I asked you if you were ready to come back to this realm. You replied that you wanted to dance in the Milky Way for a while, then you would go home. I bid you "good dancing" and left you dancing among the stars.

Dylan's Protection Meditation

You are the shimmering, luminous universe
You are the shimmering, luminous sphere, silver-platinum
You are the shimmering, luminous collective prayers
You are the shimmering, luminous breath, the prana, of life
You are the shimmering, luminous light that supports and heals you
You are the shimmering, luminous flame that consumes negativity
You are the shimmering, luminous sword which cuts away negativity
You are the shimmering, luminous reflection
You are the shimmering, luminous universe

21 Huna Breath Process:

1. Short and seemed surprised that it was short.
2. Short and impatient that it was short.
3. Short and impatient that it was short.
4. Short . . . I said, "Dylan, be grateful for your breath."
5. Short . . . I said, "Breathe slowly through pursed lips . . . like whistling."
6. Deeper, I said, "Breathe slowly, slowly."
7. Deeper, I said, "Be grateful."
8. You yawned . . . cautiously.
9. Yawned again . . . cautious again.
10. - 16. A shift. Breaths became about two-thirds full.
17. Shorter, due to tiredness.
18. Same as 17. I told Dylan that I was going to put my hands on his lungs, front and back and my hands would follow the rise and fall of his breath.
19. You yawned fairly deeply . . . no pain!
20. Sighed and said, "I am sleepy now."
21. Sighed deeply. I said, "You sleep, I will keep breathing for you!"

The next 21 varied but overall were distinctively deeper and similar to ten through sixteen's two-thirds breath, which I was glad to see! I kept my hands on his lungs during this process.

Good evening, Dylan,

I have been tuning into you all day. A lot of lightness still prevails. In a dream I had this afternoon I saw you floating and flying around in the air. You seemed very much in control of your movements and enjoying being in control.

For my part, after the protection and during the meditation, I just keep getting a lot of lightness and tenderness. TLC, if you will. For the time being I am carrying you around on a satin pillow . . . a blue one. It has white ribbons on the corners that float and fly with you. During the healing a lot of lightness permeates your being and the healing process. It seems that just the mildest touch accomplishes a lot. Just the touch of my fingertips brings a notice to your body, mind and spirit. You are so tuned into life, Dylan. So tuned in.

Basically, the intent is that you do no work . . . just accept and receive the healings. Let them in to the fullest extent . . . and more. I am guided by your higher self as to what direction the healing process takes. I have no thought or position to take any control of this process. I am a vehicle or a conduit for this energy and your higher self instructs me as to which modality we address.

Tonight I stood on my tiptoes and lifted you as high as I could into the air, with you resting on your blue satin pillow, the ribbons waving in the breeze. First the sun, in a setting stage, filled you with Sun energy, brilliantly and colorfully energizing you. Then, the full moon appeared, and embraced and enfolded you in its sweet and gentle mellowness. The stars added their sparkle in their own special manner and the Milky Way glowed brightly just for you. You are blessed by the heavens, Dylan. I am sure this pleases your mystical and artistic nature.

Then, I lowered my arms and placed you on green grass, fresh from today's rain. The raindrops fell from the tree branches, dancing droplets falling on your face. You loved it! All the green energy from the trees and the grass blended together with the sun, moon and star energy to complement the healing. As above, so below, Dylan. I added extra fresh Reiki green energy bandage inside and outside your tender body. I then placed you back on your satin pillow. Sleep well, my precious prince.

Dear Dylan,

"Do you know where you're going to? Do you like the things that life is showing you? Where are you going to . . . do you know?"

Again, Dylan, as last night, and a few other times here and there, I am finding you with one foot here and one foot there. I also see you lifting in and out of your body as if you were "trying on" the other side. I can also see you as transparent. The other side has no pain, but it does have a conscious sense of loss and a void from this view. It is natural to want to know what is over there. What you have to measure is what you will lose and what you will gain.

The green Reiki bandage is wrapped from your head to your feet, securely keeping you supplied with healing energy. The Great China Wall is surrounding your lungs. A smaller wall, but just as strong, is behind your left knee. That area has been taking a lot of energy as well. The mitochondria are gathered in great numbers in your lungs and in your left leg. They are charged with energy to support you in life. The grid is strong and in its formal design, not curving to form around your torso. The protection method is impenetrable.

Even though Dianne Carroll's words came at the beginning, I am hearing Mozart now, as I did the night I gave you a bath. Classical music, Mozart, would be great to listen to . . . especially with an accompaniment by James Galway, the flutist. Ahhhh . . . very healing.

Be good to yourself, Dylan. Strong name, strong man, be strong, be very strong. Goodnight.

Dearest tender soldier,

Everything is written. We all have our own script. We do not stay up late to study and memorize our lines. Our lines, embodied in our thoughts, actions and words lead, guide and move us through each moment, each day and each measure of time. We are in charge of little and of everything.

Some creations are born with "additional" organs and systems. Some have several hearts, several stomachs and just different physiological designs. I sense this with you, Dylan. Physically you have the design of any human on the planet, but you also have other bodies, some seen and some unseen, that have extended organs and systems. I perceive that you are dancing the intricate steps of discovering your other bodies. You feel that you are on the dance floor alone, but at times, a Great Presence is revealed to you.

This Great Presence reads your script to you. Then you know . . . you know without knowing. On the "invisible" plane you know everything. Everything that has happened with you, from the beginning of time, at this moment and in the future. You have the liberty, the freedom, to move from one world into another and back again. The other worlds mirror your other bodies as you dance to the music of your script.

Later, I asked you to take a walk with me. It was a nature walk with fields, flowers and trees. There was one tree, one particular tree, standing alone in the field. It was on a slight hill, just above us. You started to stride determinedly toward the tree, going ahead of me. I slowed my steps to watch you march. When you reached the tree, you did not stop . . . you walked, without hesitation, into the tree. You allowed me to "see" you inside the tree trunk. You stood for a while, in the broad trunk. You invited the sturdiness and strength of the tree into your body. You stayed in that space of receiving for another while, absorbing the life, the juices, of the tree. You were between breaths, between time and space, and between worlds.

Suddenly, your eyes blinked open wide. You became fascinated with the tree! You began counting the rings in the trunk. Then, you stretched your feet down into the roots. You put your head back and looked up into the limbs and extended your head and arms into the tallest branches. You laughed uproariously! You thought this was a major cool happening. Becoming one with the tree, you counted the rings in the branches. Now, focusing on your own trunk you counted your rings on down into your feet, then up to your head, arms and hands. A wise being, so mystical, studying the tiers of life. Afterwards, you moved your whole body up to the top branches and shouted that you could see a long way off.

I sat on the ground and waited for you.

Lilly said, "I touched him. I touched him today."

It was as if the Lord God sent all his angels singing those words. I exclaimed, "What? You touched him? Thank you, God, thank you, God!"

Lilly said, "I touched him on his back, behind his heart, and also on his head. I did the Reiki and was going to do something else but didn't."

I was exuberant, exhilarated, celebrating a movement into the process. Lilly was rewarded for making a decision to find her voice and speak her truth. She didn't see that at first . . . I saw it clearly, Lilly was rewarded for her decision.

I am sensing a quiet, sleepy house over there. No nausea, but hungry. Knocked out with exhaustion and shock to system. Very quiet. Reiki is outside his body, packed around his tender form and filling his room. Reiki inside his body is vibrating and shooting around in laserlike fashion. It is as if the Reiki is trying to hit all the important places at once and all the places are important. There is also a "dodge ball" game with the Reiki trying to dodge the chemo and radiation impact. The chemo and radiation are rampant, going to and fro, mixing, tumbling, power plays, juggling for position. Reiki is the overseer, the watchdog, making sure each goes where it is supposed to, all the while staying out of target's way. Dad is scared, wants to run to Mother and cry in her lap. "My son, my son, what am I going to do? I can do anything but I cannot help my son!" Neither Mom nor Dad can turn to each other for solace. That left a long time ago. Unfortunate. Dad does have his parents. Mom's passed away. Poor Liam, the oldest and only other child, booted with Dylan's birth and now has to justify all his resentful childhood feelings and coordinate them with the current adult caregiving and grief.

We are all worried about Lilly. She does have an older sister, Sandy. Her sister keeps her distance, maybe more than she ordinarily would. Lilly has been so dismissed and discounted in this family. Probably more since her adoring parents left her.

From midnight to 2 A.M. I sent Reiki to Dylan. I held his head, top, back, face for an hour. I whispered in his ear, "It is okay, it is all right, everything is okay, it is all right," over and over. I smoothed the etheric energy over his face until it was relaxed. His eyes under his eyelids stopped racing. His jaw lowered, he turned his head to the side for sleep. I put my hands over his chest, not going inside the lungs to disturb the process, the blending of the samariam radioisotopes and the gymsidobine, just to allow the process to be more peaceful and easier for Dylan.

At 3:58 A.M. I was awakened by his energy. His heart seemed to be racing and he was panicking. I was guided to give him the Reiki Professional Degree initiation. The instant that energy was in him it began racing from his head to his toes and back again, over and over; so fast. I asked the energy why it was rushing so quickly in this manner. The energy replied, "There is so much to do, we have to move quickly!" I know that Reiki has its own innate, Divine intelligence. I moved back to Dylan's head and placed my hands there until he calmed again.

He seemed to be awake again at 6 A.M. and again at 8 A.M. I knew the Home Health nurse was coming between 8 and 8:30 to draw blood to check his hemoglobin count. It was 8.9—14-15 is optimum. He will go for more transfusions today. His heart rate was 117, still racing. Lilly is wondering about Dylan breathing through his mouth and if it is lowering the benefit of the oxygen tubes in his nose. The nurse noted that Dylan's blood was thin and asked if he was on blood thinners because his blood was having difficulty clotting. The blend of the radiation and the chemotherapy will lower his platelets to the degree that he will have to have those transfusions also. Lilly called around 10:30 A.M., said Dylan was really "out," eyelids could not open, labored breathing and there were spaces between his breaths. I said, "Om Namah Shivaya."

Yesterday, Lilly said that two computers were out and the maid had a sore throat. She asked me if I knew what that might mean. Later, I did a reading on that. The reading said that there were "short-circuited personalities in the house and the maid was sick because she was sad about what was going on in the house." Lilly is very lovely. It was clear that when they got home Dad would take the jealous anger out on her, possibly accusing her of flirting with the one who complimented her. I really hesitated to tell Lilly the results of the reading; it felt invasive and private. However, she wants to know, so I related it to her.

She said, "Foreign."

I said, "I beg your pardon?"

"He was born where women are subservient," she said quietly.

Now, so much made sense. Her being dismissed and discounted in her house, having no voice, no respect. He was not allowing her to even exist!

Around noon my left hand felt like it was going to come off. That is where I had his head (with the rest of his body in my left arm). It was reflecting the fall I am sure. I almost told Lilly today that when he went in for blood work to call an ambulance so he could lie down for the trip, but he went for another reason.

Lilly just called and said that about noon Dylan fell and hit his head. He was brought to the emergency room by ambulance, given an MRI, which was clear. The impact was on his left cheekbone. He was given two units of blood, waited for the hemoglobin count and was told to have a third unit of blood. They plan to be home about 1:30.

When she called a moment ago I did not recall the above information, but after she told me I remembered. I also told her it was hard for me to find him and asked if they were going to admit him. She answered no—the doctors said the new medication would kick in next week. I pray so.

It is difficult to tell what the lessons are for all of us involved. I am grateful to God for the lessons and know that infinite wisdom is working through all.

After Lilly's call last night around 10:15, I began to work on her, in addition to Dylan. For some reason it was difficult to find him . . . possibly all the machines . . . and I had a fever. He was still in my left hand and arm, "lightly." I used my right hand for Lilly and put it on her head, face and neck, then over her heart and later over her adrenal glands in her back. I did the 21-breath process, and also did the breath on each of her chakras to boost her. She absorbed the energy like a dry sponge in water. After a while I gave her an absent "hug" and installed her in my right hand and arm, then focused again on Dylan.

He is so very light and weak. His symptoms of spaces between breaths, not opening his eyes, or his eyes not focusing concern me greatly. Bless his princely heart. I was encouraged that the doctors said the new medicine would take effect next week. He continues to absorb and desire the Reiki. Thank goodness, left brain-wise, I have the clinical research studies that have proven Reiki to boost the immune system, lower pain and stabilize blood pressure, etc. I feel sad for Lilly and for me, that a "miracle" has not yet happened with the Reiki . . . or at least one that I would recognize that way.

I always begin with my hands on his precious head, to calm him. Then I scan his whole body and see what triggers the energy, and I go to that spot. His heart is handling a lot of the side effects of the treatments . . . I am so glad he is young and has a strong heart. I next breathe for him . . . sometimes it feels like I am the only one breathing. I do the breaths slowly and long. I am glad when I sense a connection with our breaths. Then I do the breath for his blood to introduce oxygen into it. I visualize the balance of the appropriate number of red and white blood cells. I did the breath on each of his chakras, or energy centers. Next I go to his heart and thank it profusely for the work it is doing. I inform his heart how important it is to his body and that we all are grateful for it being so strong when he needs it so much. I address the mitochondria in the cells to be as active as they can with the onslaught of the medicine affecting them. I do the breath for them until I see them moving actively.

I end by calming him again, over all his body . . . part of this is the protection spheres, part of this is wrapping his body in the Reiki green bandage. Much of it is pure prayer for his suffering to be relieved and for healing his body, mind and spirit. I also include prayers for the whole family for the support of Dylan's wellness and balance and harmony in the home.

Then, I put Dylan back into my left arm and hand. His head and neck are in my hand, upper torso up to the elbow, then lower torso and feet up to my shoulder. I even felt him tickle my ear with his toes . . . he does have humor! I also took that to indicate a foot rub would be a good idea, so I did that.

Report:
Left calf hurts. Scared of not being able to get a breath. Wake up in fear of this. Dread of doctors and treatments. Also grateful to Julia. Sadness . . . want a

girlfriend I can keep. Want my mother relieved. Want it over. Lost my father. Can't run to him. Out of breath trying. Need to let him go. Let everybody go and just be myself. Money . . . who is going to pay for me? Need more clothes to wear. Love my mother's cooking. I like chicken. I want to go home. I want a pain group. I love my dog. Say a prayer for me. Warmth in head . . . relaxes neck muscles, helps headache. Releases tension in upper chest . . . lungs . . . going lower . . . easier to breathe . . . eases fear. Relaxation out shoulders, down arms to hands, down body, through legs, extra warm on painful left leg. Relaxed down to feet. Deeper relaxation in mediastinum and on down to solar plexsus. Filled up like a balloon with Reiki. Feel better. More relaxing in upper respiratory. All breathing relaxes. A little dread still at the bottom of lungs. Ok. Better. Throat relaxes. Less awareness of pain. Wants children.

I last heard from Lilly yesterday at 1:30 P.M. It is now 24 hours since. My intuition tells me to wait for her call. She knows the class was devoted to him and she usually wants to know any reports. I hope everything is all right, that he is still here. I can feel him in my hands.

I did reach Lilly later, around 5 P.M. She was resting, but she said she was not sleeping and was thinking about me. She related bizarre crises that occurred during the night. The oxygen tanks were not working. Dylan's nose was bleeding . . . a water soluble lotion was put into his nostrils . . . oil should not be mixed with oxygen. Dylan is totally in charge of his many medications and takes whatever he wants, whenever he wants.

Lilly said, "Julia, Dylan asked me to hold his hand." I was so moved, so proud of him, so happy for her. I said quietly, "Thank you, God." She said that when he asked her she was sitting on the floor by his bed. She sat on the floor for a long time and then asked someone to get her a chair, but she did not let go of her son's hand. She said she did Reiki on him with every breath. I reminded her that when she had to carry him, full body weight, several times, in the hospital, how precious it was to do that for her son. She replied that it was the best experience a mother could have. She is little and he is over six feet tall . . . and she carried him.

Today, around 3 P.M., I called to see how things were going. Last night I sent an email about a concern for a ministroke and a possible roving clot. I also mentioned the improbability of that with his thin blood. Lilly informed me just how thin it was. They were in a hurry, leaving for the hospital for a platelet transfusion. Taking a deep breath, I inquired as to what the platelet count was. "Ten," she answered. I couldn't respond. After a while, I repeated, "Ten?" Ten thousand. I drew a deeper breath, really deep. Normal platelet count is 250,000. I knew the radiation and chemo would gobble them up, but not to that degree.

It is almost 1 A.M. now. I am wondering if they are home.

Lilly called around 11 A.M. and said that there were four people taking care of Dylan around the clock. That he was highly agitated and not sleeping. He cannot bear the oxygen mask on his face and she is amazed at his strength in trying to remove it. She has had some good conversations with him. He asked her why there was so much pain in the world. She responded that there was also a lot of love in the world.

Lily is sleeping on the floor in his room. I am so relieved that she is doing that, for herself and for him. I had imaged her sleeping on the floor outside his door a long time ago. This is better.

I did a situational absent healing for the house and all its occupants. I drew the house, put the address, named all the family members. Then did the Reiki on it. I put the drawing on my altar for a day and a night. Hopefully some harmony filled the house.

Saw Dylan in a green grass yard, jumping on a trampoline.
"I'm jumping on a trampoline, I'm jumping on a trampoline."
"See how high I can jump?"
"Look at me, look at me jump!" "I am flying, jumping and flying."
"Wheeeee."
"The sky is so blue."
"I am so high."
"Wheeeee."
I ask, "What is happening, Dylan?"
"Very little of me working now. I don't know what to do. There are many things to say, many things to be said.

"I love my mother. She is so sweet. She loves me, too. I hurt so much. I hurt all over.

"I'm glad you shook ol' Dad up.
"Mom will speak up one day, when the time is ripe."
Anything else, Dylan?
"Not now."
I filled the room with Reiki, surrounded his bed with Reiki, poured liquid Reiki into his head and it filled him all the way down to his feet.

He said it was cool and nice.

He said that sometimes his body was hot and sometimes it was really cold.

I lifted the aura over his lungs, which, in turn, allowed his rib cage to lift. This let him breathe easier and deeper.

I filled the lungs, the area between the lungs and his rib cage, then between each rib.

The Reiki surrounded his heart, cushioning it, buffering it, protecting it.

I asked all parts of his body where it wanted Reiki. Confusion reigned, everywhere.

The cells are battered.

I just filled it all . . . whole body, with liquid Reiki.

Then wrapped his body with thick Reiki bandage outside.

I kissed his forehead.

I told him that I loved him very much.

I asked him what he wanted me to do.

He replied, "The same."

I asked, "Same?"

He said, "More."

I wrapped Lilly in the green bandage. What a warrior she is. She is reaping many blessings with her son now.

She is pure love, thank goodness.

It is her strength.

Lilly called today. Dylan has not slept in two days and nights. His jaw is trembling. His eyes are staring and glazed.

Last night, he said, "Mom, this is a ship to shore call. Do you know what I mean?"

Lilly answered, "I understand."

He came and stood by my bed last night. Said he wanted to visit and tell me thank you.

Lilly saw either him on a ship or his bed was a ship or a boat. Some man was at the end of his bed holding his feet to keep him from going.

I got that Lilly was "keeping watch" last night. I also got the word "vigil." She slept on the floor in his room. I hope she does the same tonight.

Lilly also experienced Dylan asking for liquid Reiki to be poured into the top of his head, which she did. He also wanted glasses of liquid Reiki to drink and guzzled them down. When it was time for her to "close" he did not want her to go. She stayed longer, then closed. She called me and said he wanted her to stay and what did I do when he wanted that. I replied that I never close . . . he is with me all the time.

Lilly telephoned to report that Dylan's eyes are mostly open, staring and glazed. I asked if she was using some "tears" to moisten his eyes. She said he blinked enough for that need. She had talked to several physicians regarding Dylan's mouth and facial tremors. The doctors say that some medications can cause such symptoms. Dylan had some night terror between 2 and 3 A.M. . . . thinking a predator or predators had come in his door . . . one an elderly gentleman . . . to harm him.

I will tell Lilly to do Reiki on his head for his eyes to calm and hopefully close. I will ask her if his mouth is also open in an awkward way. The Reiki on his head should calm his mouth also.

I will also ask Lilly to keep a candle burning somewhere in the house possibly near Quan Yin, from 7 P.M. to 7 A.M. at least. This is his beacon when he astrally travels, in addition to the Reiki line or anchor. Interesting "boat" or "ship" terms being used.

This afternoon I put the Reiki II symbols on Dylan's third eye from mine (I frequently reinforce them during the day). The symbols were so alive and he took them and sent them forcefully down to his feet . . . as if he couldn't do it fast enough. It was as if the symbols could have been held in one's hands . . . they were so tangible. I filled his body with the emerald green Reiki liquid, checked his "line," and filled several glasses with Reiki liquid for him to drink, which he did, one after another . . . about 5-7 glasses.

I passed in front of their house at 10 A.M. this morning. The house had a silent, sleep aura. All curtains were drawn except for vertical blinds downstairs on the chimney side. Later that evening I felt very restless and was pacing around my house. At 7 P.M. I drove over to his house and passed by three times, parked and sent energy to the house, especially to his room. I saw a huge flash of light suddenly shooting from the roof. I wondered if this was his conduit for astral travel. Evening outside lights were all around . . . excellent. I wondered if they were on all night. A bright light enhanced the red door entrance . . . superb. Dylan needs tangible ways to find his way home when he travels. After awhile I drove home.

I arrived home, wanting so very much to call Lilly. Something made me wait and at 10:20 P.M., she called.

She softly and waveringly said, "My dear Julia, our precious son left us tonight, and they just picked up his body."

I was stunned and asked at what time. She said at 7:15. I replied that I had been in front of the house at that time. I asked her for her permission to keep working with him.

She said, "Take Dylan to the brightest light." I told Lilly that I loved her and would do as she requested. He left his body while I was sitting in front of his house. Totally amazing. I wonder if that was him, that flash of light.

Lilly sent me a sweet email calling me Dylan's spiritual companion and wanting me to continue his reports.

Last night I emailed Lilly to have a candle burning until dawn if possible. I sensed Dylan was mostly at his mother's last night. He was with me some. He wanted to know the Reiki II symbols, said I did not teach them to him and wanted to know if there were additional symbols for the Professional Degree. No additional ones.

Lilly called today at 1:40 P.M. and left a message. Her voice was barely present. She said she was calling for no special reason, just to thank me for my constant vigilance with Dylan. Lilly called back at 4:45 P.M. Sounded very down. She said until today it was as if he was off on a trip, but she realized today that he was really gone and would not be back. She asked a lot of questions about what form he was in now, and when he totally merged with the light, wouldn't he be one with everything?

The planets aligned positively this afternoon and I felt compelled to do the ceremony at Dylan's gravesite. I went there today with a silver bowl that contained Thai Jasmine rice, Sandalwood oil, amber powder, kumkum, Sacred Ash from a Yagna, rose petals from his service, some soil from his grave and the appropriate Mantras. It was very moving, a closure for me and for Dylan. I put the mixture at his crown, third eye, throat, heart, solar and sacral plexuses and base of his spine, then at his hands, knees and feet. I sprinkled the remainder over all the rest of his body's resting place. I stood at his head and talked to him, thanking him for the friendship, wishing him Godspeed on his journey and telling him he could go now. It is the eve of a new moon and it is the eve of Diwali, a New Year I celebrate. Goodbye, my Prince. I love you. I thank you for this journey with you.

I felt compelled to go to Dylan's gravesite again. I had the small statuette of a little Prince and felt I should take it there. The statue had his hand over his heart and the other hand extended out as if he was giving love from his heart. I drove there, parked, went through the hedge and walked up the sidewalk toward his place of rest. My eye caught on a brilliantly yellow star-shaped leaf just before his grave. I was instantly reminded of the tiny gold star by the feather at my door the other night. I did not pick up the leaf, just thanked it for whatever the message was. As I got to the plot I first checked to see if the mounds of special rice were there . . . all there . . . exactly in place. I took the Prince statue and dug a little hole just above the crown chakra area and placed it there. It looked very regal and natural. I chanted some mantras, knelt and observed the energy to see what, if anything, I could intuit. Everything felt peaceful and at ease. I was just beginning to walk around the site three times and the Little Prince said, "You should put a coin under me." I pulled a shiny dime from my pocket, lifted the Little Prince out of the dirt, put the dime under it, and secured it into the dirt again. There were some loose white rose petals from Dylan's service that I had sprinkled around with the rice. I took some and made a circle of rose petals around the Little Prince. Then, surveying the energy again, I stood at Dylan's head area and walked around the site, clockwise three times, saying Mantras as I went. I knelt again and waited to see if anything else would reveal itself. And, felt nothing. I walked backwards away from the grave, as one always does with a high being, then turned around to go to my car. As I turned around the bright yellow leaf seemed to say, "So long, see you next time." I still thought perhaps I should take it, just to have it, but left it, for next time.

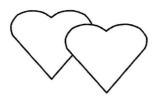

STOMACH
Anne

The phone in my office rings at least three times a week with an announcement that a diagnosis of cancer has just been received by a client.

There is no way that I have found to prepare myself for these phone calls. Once, a physician who referred clients to me, asked me why my phone did not ring for sprained ankles, tennis elbow and common colds. I had no answer for that, just that it appears my karma is to work with the catastrophic illnesses. Many do not experience the terminal category, but some do. Death is a healing also.

A friend of a friend asked that I treat Anne, who had been diagnosed with an extremely rare form of stomach cancer. Anne was in her midseventies, was married, had four grown children and had an active social and business life. She was well known and well loved in the community. I had done some real estate business with her in the past and knew her to be an astute businessperson with high integrity.

The doctors at the cancer hospital had sent Anne home saying there was nothing more they could do. Anne's family felt otherwise and therefore telephoned me.

I frequently go to hospitals and homes when the individual is unable to come to my office. With flowers and a sweet card in my hands, I rang the doorbell. The last time I had seen Anne was in her real estate office where her energy and charm filled the room. This time was different. Her husband and daughter walked me into the bedroom and I saw a very ill and very weak elderly lady. She could not lift her head or say very much at all. Her husband helped me set up the Reiki treatment table at the end of her bed. Before the treatment he assisted her to the bathroom and held her so she would not fall. He then more than half carried her and placed her on the treatment table. Her full head of hair, always perfect and attractive, was now spare and fuzzy, like a newborn's.

When pillows and blankets were arranged I began the treatment by touching her head to promote relaxation and give her a sense of how Reiki felt. She was so very weak and fell right to sleep. Anne was on heavy doses of morphine along with chemotherapy. So, sleep was a gift.

After the treatment, Will lifted her, sweetly and gently, and placed her back into bed. He set up a twenty-one-day treatment session, which is the norm for cancer or a serious situation.

Everyday for about a week, the situation was the same as the first day. Anne could not lift her head, had to be carried to the treatment table, was heavily medicated and also was not eating anything at all. It appeared that the end was very close.

After the first week, Will answered the door with a big smile on his face. I had trained him in Reiki also and he had been treating his wife diligently in my absence. Anne was sitting up. She had eaten some strawberries and a little piece of a muffin. Will was ecstatic. So was I! I entered her room quietly as usual, still expecting to see a nonresponsive patient listlessly lying in the bed. Not this time. She was not only sitting up, she got up, went to the toilet by herself and literally hopped upon the Reiki table. She was smiling and chatting away. A different Anne, for sure. The entire week was like this and Anne even attended, in a wheelchair, a Bar Mitzvah for her grandnephew. No one could believe it, not even Anne.

Now, Anne had lived a full life, and in her view, not a very happy one. It had been difficult raising four children and she had been widowed once, too. During this widowhood she started a business from scratch and became very successful. She felt she had no choice. She had to survive and provide for her children. A piano sat in the parlor but she never had time to play. There was a state-of-the-art kitchen but she never had time to cook. Her home and gardens were picture perfect but she never had time to entertain. She was not happy.

She could not "stomach" her life. And her stomach got the message.

Suddenly, Anne realized that she was getting better. She did enjoy all the attention from me and everyone but this was not her plan. She wanted to leave. She wanted to rest. She wanted to have at least one thing in her life go her way. No one was going to take it away from her. She informed her husband that she had a new and different pain and wanted to return to the cancer hospital. This set everyone back. Was the Reiki now not working? Had the Reiki caused something to happen inside her body? What was this development?

The doctors all knew Anne very well by this time. They did more tests, more x-rays, ultrasounds and administered more medicines through the intravenous tubes. I was there every day. Anne sweetly introduced me to her nurses and doctors. She had readjusted her plan and I was no longer a threat. Hospice came in and Anne readily agreed to sign up with them. Hospice caretakers, angels on earth, only enter the scene when the patient has less than six months to live. With Anne it was determined that it would be much shorter.

Anne was taken home. The twenty-one-day Reiki treatment plan still had another week to go. Anne was getting out of bed and able to get onto the treatment table. Each day while Anne was receiving her treatment, she inquired, "Is today the twenty-first day?" I asked her if she would like for it to be the twenty-first day. She smiled and insisted that she wanted her full twenty-one days. Her husband and daughter already had planned on another twenty-one-day plan, but I knew Anne had something else in mind. Her death. Each day, Anne would repeat her question, "Is today the twenty-first day?" And, each day, I would answer, "Would you like for it to be the twenty-first day?"

For the last three or four treatment days I observed that Anne had less and less energy. She asked me if she was going to live. I told her that it was up to her. The energy in her stomach had leveled out and was very responsive to the Reiki. I said that she knew all she had accomplished the last three weeks and it was up to her to continue with activities or not. She held my face and said, "You have such a beautiful face, like an angel's." She said that she would not continue with another twenty-one days, that she was ready to go to God. She said that she knew her husband, children and grandchildren would miss her dearly, but this was life and it was time for her to go. She thanked me so very much for all I had done and wished me well in my work. Anne said that people were lucky if they got to experience my work and she knew she was leaving a different person because of the Reiki. It was sad to say goodbye for both of us. She had asked for a photo of me and kept it on her bedside table.

For the next four weeks, I sent flowers, then cards, then telephoned and finally stopped all contact. After another month I called to see how she was and Will said she had just peacefully passed away in her sleep. He said she was in no pain and had been taking no medications at all for over a month. I was very glad to hear that. He said he knew the Reiki gave her an elevated quality of life and peace before she left, but he also acknowledged that she wanted to go. We all miss her and think of her looking down upon us with her gracious smile. We feel now she has time to play her piano, to cook and entertain in her fragrant garden. Goodbye, Dear Anne.

LEGS, ANKLES and FEET
Julia, Adrienne and Amanda

When God created man, God said, "Let man walk." Well, I am sure God said something like that somewhere. Anyway, it fits here.

I do believe that soon after I was born I started running, running and running. There was never a time in which I chose to be still, so I ran. I ran as a toddler, from room to room in the house. As a schoolgirl I won all the events that required speed. As a teenager I ran from boyfriend to boyfriend. And, in college I raced through all the courses and couldn't go fast enough. Four days after college graduation I raced into marriage and quickly raced out of it, twice. I sped through motherhood and several careers. My life took turn after turn with hints and clues for me to slow down and look at my life, to see what I was rocketing through. But I kept on; fast life, fast cars, fast airplanes, fast money.

One day another speeder, in a car, hit my car. I had many injuries and was in rehabilitation for almost a year. The crucial injury was my left leg. *Note:* we kneel to God with our right leg and we kneel to man with our left leg. My left leg was wrapped around the steering wheel and pinned to the dashboard.

There was glass and metal everywhere, and soon the ambulances and police vehicles surrounded me. I heard my meditation Mantra, and it stilled and calmed me. Then my mind began to spin; I had my daughter's car. I thought how I could break this news to her and how rapidly I could replace Mandy's prized sports car. All the while the first responders were doing their job, prying off the door, untangling my limbs and wiping blood away to check for any major bleeders. I began to fire swift questions at the paramedics and police. "What is your name, who hit me, did he have insurance, which hospital are you taking me to?"

At the hospital, on a gurney, not quite conscious, I asked the time. It was 4:55 P.M. and it was a Friday. The offices would be closed all weekend, and it was five minutes before my insurance office closed. I wanted to act quickly: telephone my agent, lease a car, call my attorney and notify Mandy to come and get me. I demanded a phone be brought to me right away. A nurse gently informed me that I was too injured to take time for calls and I must get to the x-ray room and then to surgery. Even with all this I did not slow down. Again I insisted on a phone, and the nurse wheeled the gurney to a counter so I could make my calls. She had to dial and for some reason I did not notice that I could not.

I reached everyone, dictating instructions with rapid-fire hysteria. After that the nurse, looking relieved and somewhat in awe of my actions, wheeled me into the examining room. It is amazing what can be done when one is in shock. The Mantra was droning in my ears.

In the process of the examinations and x-rays, the pain began to creep in. I do not remember much about this part. I do recall asking all the doctors their names and specialties. I also thought I was completely coherent and was later told that I was babbling nonsense. The ambulance came and moved me to another hospital and another steady stream of doctors, radiologists, neuropsychologists, endodontists, rehabilitation teams and many others. Within the walls of the hospital I was again racing, from one doctor to another with more examinations, x-rays and tests. In all this activity, I kept hearing the physicians say, "watch that leg or go slow with that leg." After a few weeks, the medical team was still cautious and careful with my left leg. There were other injuries and it appeared that the leg would be addressed in a "last but not least" fashion.

My leg was mangled and twisted and many devices were designed to accommodate it. For what seemed forever it was elevated and in traction, plus being encased in ice. There were various casts, then braces, then crutches combined with the braces. Meanwhile, I was feeling active and wanted to be discharged.

Five months had passed; I had lots to make up for and lots to do for the future. I seemed to be the only one concerned about that. To say that I was a difficult patient is an understatement. My life was on jet planes to the tune of a hundred thousand miles each year. I had gone from a warp-speed life to, in my mind, a dead stop. Four doctors did state that I should not have lived through this. I thought that a few of them secretly wished I hadn't. I was a very angry lady. Luckily, I had my Mantra to soothe and to comfort me.

Finally, surgery was approved for my leg. The other injuries were either healed or under control. The doctor was very reputable and I trusted him completely. I requested, and was granted, a headset so I could listen to my Mantra during the surgery. I also requested that the doctors make only positive statements during the surgery and not listen to any heavy metal or rock music, either. I asked my daughter to please have the Mantra playing in my room when I was brought out of surgery.

I slept heavily for the first day. Breathing machines, physical therapists, and many doctors were in and out. (The phrase I heard most was, "no weight on that leg." Another therapist came in to teach me how to walk, how to take care of still another cast, and to give me instructions regarding elevation and icing the leg.)

On the third day, my daughter and a good friend brought me home. Yay, no ambulance this time. I was experiencing pain, aggravation and impatience. The cast, crutches and other apparatus were cumbersome and awkward. There were more icepacks, more elevations, more bed rest and, unbelievably, more physical therapy for four to five days each week.

I lay there, day after day, week after week wondering what on earth, besides slowing down, was the lesson in all this. Each time the answer was just that; to slow down. Nowhere in my mindset was an understanding of slowing down. I kept thinking I could function but family and friends were quick to assure me otherwise. I watched spiritual videos all day, everyday. My favorites were stories of the *Bhagavad Gita* and the mystical, ancient music of India.

I still could not bend the left leg at all. The "description" was a shelf resection, which was reshaping the femur to fit the tibia and fibula. This is basically connecting the "leg bones to the hip bone." A chronoplasty was performed, as well as a procedure to remove debris from the internal derangement and a serious miniscus repair. After a month the doctors said we could begin some aggressive rehabilitation.

The rehabilitation began—four days a week for an hour or more each time. For about a month many therapies were utilized, including a tub whirlpool, large pool exercises, ultrasound, medication patches and various touch therapies. One day I walked in and the therapist said, "Okay, today we try to bend the knee." The tears in my eyes were from fear, gratitude or both. She took my foot, lifted it and bent the knee a half-inch or so. The pain was like a hot knife searing through my atrophied leg. She quickly said, "That's enough for today." It was a miniscule movement but I felt a sense of achievement. Several more visits encouraged more measures of movement. Each time the techniques and achievements were recorded. After another two months the temporary cast could be permanently removed and weight could be applied. This was monumental. I acquired many nicknames along this wellness path; "Festus, Chester, Gimpy-Limpy," and other endearing and attractive labels. My Mantra supported me through all this.

As I could apply weight I realized that I would now have to lift my entire left side. My left shoulder, followed by the left hip, must all lift together in order for me to raise and swing my leg forward for one step. The leg and foot were basically rigid. After a while, I attempted lifting the top half of my leg so the knee would bend naturally. That worked for the leg and knee. It's just that the foot did not know what to do. It was unbending. This idea was not completely working, so I had to rethink my process. For seven months, my whole left side had been drawn up due to inactivity. It was an entirely new education process.

I realized, suddenly, painfully and very fearfully, that I could not walk. Running, swimming and jumping, skiing, hiking up mountains, bike riding and the like became something I "used to do." Friends teased me because they did not know what else to do. Other friends just left me for the same reason. My exercises became my driving force. I could not walk or drive so I was dependent on any and all resources. My day was divided into therapy, exercises and a lot of meditation. Work was out of the question.

Reaching for my foot, which felt like a foreign object, trying to dress or to tie a shoe became major time consumers. I would look at my foot as if it did not belong to me. My daughter and friends were my cheerleaders and supported every tiny achievement, and they were all tiny. With lessened pain, my mind was clearer. I began to mentally communicate with my leg and foot. I asked them to forgive me for rushing around and hurrying through life. I mentally connected the part of my body that did work with the part of my body that did not work. I would ask these separate parts to work together, to communicate and to teach the nonworking side to work. The Mantra was forever and steadfastly playing. It was my biggest support.

As the guided meditations, combined with all the rehabilitations, began to pay off, I recognized that I must honor my body—all the bodies; the physical, the mental and the spiritual. I perceived this situation as a gift from God and a wake-up call to change my life. I realized that I was not racing around the globe to work, but that I was running to escape life. In my consciousness, I was never where I was. I was always in the next place or the next place after that. I was not living in the present.

I learned that my body was my temple created by God and that it must be honored.

I am eternally grateful to the Mantra for being my lifeline, for being my constant companion, for teaching me the stillness within and incorporating the knowledge that it will always be my reverent source. I give thanks above all, to my Guru, for it is She who gave me the Mantra.

Adrienne

I am in no way an astrologer, but I do know that all the ancient sages and holy beings were educated in astrology. Even policemen, doctors and school principals cringe when it is a full moon. There are statistically more crimes, more injuries and more events of mischievousness with a full moon. Go ahead, if you like, and blame the politicians for the economy and wars; blame the airline pilots and ship captains for accidents, but it is the stars. The stars go in cycles as do the people and events.

Now, what does this have to do with ankles and feet? Everything.

The two following case histories are indications of a first and second Saturn return. Saturn is a planet that demands regulations, rules and structure. Saturn returns occur between our twenty-seventh and twenty-ninth year, again between our fifty-seventh and fifty-ninth year and yet again between our eighty-seventh and our eighty-ninth year. It usually affects the structure in our life and we radically change our life during this time. When I was twenty-eight I moved from New England to the Deep South, got a divorce and began a new career. Another friend got married and moved to Europe. At times our bones are literally affected. Saturn is the ruler of the structure of our inner universe and can alter them in order for us to walk a different path.

Adrienne was twenty-nine years old. She had moved from New England to the West Coast. She was in love and was also pursuing some advanced educational endeavors. Being on the West Coast was quite an adventure for her and she was happy and excited. Then, on a bicycle ride, she fell and broke her ankle. This was not part of her new life plan.

She was in a cast and on uncomfortable crutches for at least two months. Adrienne is a wise individual with an intelligence as well as an innate spirituality. With her introspection and philosophy background she examined this accident. She knew there was some kind of message her body was conveying to her. The question was, what was the message? Adrienne was unaware of the Saturn planetary aspects, and had a condescending view of astrology anyway. After all, it is not an exact science. Astrologers believe differently. A friend urged her to contact me for some distance energy focusing with Reiki Touch Therapy and some cell memory work to figure out the answers to her questions.

I have known Adrienne since she was a teenager and she wants every-thing precisely in its place and has to have a concrete reason for all occur-rences. She had already considered that perhaps this accident was a message for her to slow down and take life a little easier, not that she knew how to do that. Her entire life consisted of one challenge after another. She was an only child with a single mom and grew up very quickly. She made the remark that Sam, her boyfriend, was being just great about her accident. That simple remark was so much information for me.

It told me that she felt guilty that she had a broken ankle, was in pain and needed Sam's help. Any boyfriend, mother, friend or even a neighbor has com-passion for someone in pain and wants to help. So, one part of Adrienne's heal-ing process was to learn to receive while she could not be her usual frantic self.

The first thing we addressed was achieving balance. Being such a brilliant individual she had never paid much attention to her body. Adrienne did not even know how to ride a bicycle. Most young children know that, but even at twenty-nine, it was not part of her accomplishments. Again, her sports-minded boyfriend knew she could not ride a bike, yet insisted that they go bike riding! Who is this guy? Some men have to be trained to take care of a woman.

There was balance of the body and the mind to consider. Adrienne's spir-itual side is very developed, as is her intuition, so it was relatively easy to com-municate with her on those levels. Saturn was clearly grounding her so she would be forced to look at her life and make some decisions. Having to be still for two months definitely provided this opportunity. The next cell memory process revealed her brain in different boxes, designed like a maze. As I observed more closely I saw some murky, hidden places then also realized the maze had no outlets. In the hidden areas were subjects that Adrienne had neatly tucked and logically said, "I'll deal with you later." These subjects were now backing up on her and forcing her to deal with them. They were rebelling and saying, "My turn." These were deep and difficult issues that are typical of what Saturn presents to us in order to clarify our life structure and purpose. With Adrienne's nature being orderly and precise and having her work progress smoothly, it is typical to think that everything is okay. And, to actu-ally believe that she will get around to "it." Saturn provided the bicycle acci-dent and the broken ankle as a gift for her to take time for her body and also for her heart.

In one cell memory I recalled that in some areas of Tibet, when a new baby is born it is taken to an icy river. It is held by its ankles and dipped, head first into this river. The dipping is repeated several times. If the baby survives this dipping it is perceived that it will survive the rigors of the Tibetan climate and other hardships. In the meditation this was a dunking for both Adrienne and also Sam, and had a lot, if not everything, to do with this relationship. Adrienne had to learn to receive and Sam had to learn to give. It was also vital that she expected him to take care of her and vital for him to learn that he should, with great love, fulfill her needs.

Goddesses are on the planet to provide love, beauty and graciousness. Men are here to learn that. Goddesses innately can summon anything or anyone for any purpose desired. Adrienne must own and activate her goddess self and Sam must drop his macho ego and own his feminine side, too.

The meditations and healings continued with messages such as "assimilate," "stillness" and "regroup." As the ankle healed, so did Adrienne—body, mind and spirit. She eventually decided that Sam was not for her.

They remain good friends, but she realizes that it is an intellectual relationship and not one where he understands her full feminine self. Sam is not able, at this time, to surrender to compassion. Adrienne also decided that the West Coast was not for her and returned to New England where she was born. Her mother, stepfather, grandmother and other relatives are there and she has a new appreciation for family love and support. Adrienne is on a learning curve to blend this with her independent nature and her brilliant mind.

Amanda

What are feet anyway? What purpose do they serve? Many cultures have different belief systems about feet. In some parts of the Far East a surgeon will not operate on a foot because it is felt that the feet carry the karma of the individual. If the surgeon operates on the foot then the karma is not only altered, the surgeon has volunteered to personally take it on. Also in the Near East, in India and other adjoining countries, a Holy Being or Guru has his feet washed in sacred ceremonies. It is known through Christian origins that Jesus had his feet washed by his disciples.

An ancient Native American Indian saying states not to judge a man until you have walked in his moccasins. Louise Hay, a well-known positive thinking author, says that our feet are our "understanding." That we "stand" on our feet and they are "under" our body. Other metaphysicians firmly believe that our feet do carry us through life and we should honor and take particular care of them.

This is the story of Amanda. Amanda was in her second Saturn return and like Adrienne and her ankles with the first Saturn return, Amanda had some challenges with the bones in her feet. The second Saturn return can be easier due to the fact that about thirty years have passed and much wisdom has been gained. The feet at age fifty-seven to fifty-nine can also reveal the life the person has led. In this case, Amanda's feet were small, delicate, very well taken care of with obvious frequent pedicures and lots of massages with special lotions. So, what was the problem?

Numerous doctor examinations and tests over the past years had revealed that the bones had an unusual growth pattern. Part of this was from wearing the latest fashion in high heels. Another part was a very active life of dancing and trekking all over the world. Amanda was a very active person. Unfortunately, the rest of Amanda's body seemed to follow suit, and the imbalance in her feet traveled all the way up to her hip and shoulder. It became painfully obvious to her that her active life was about to take a sudden halt.

She called me and asked if I would consider accepting her as a client. If possible she really wanted to avoid surgery and thought perhaps Reiki Touch Therapy could prevent the surgery. I did not know if Reiki would do that but I did know that Reiki would lessen the pain and provide Amanda with peace and harmony in her body, mind and spirit. She is a sensitive soul, a lover of music and devoted to God. She is a very responsible and caring mother of two wonderful sons. There appeared to be a willingness to increase her awareness and gain more understanding about herself and life in general. I accepted Amanda as a client. I require all clients to take the first course of Reiki in order to have the ability and the responsibility to maintain the energy between appointments. Amanda was more than happy to self-treat and, over time, trained in all the levels of Reiki Touch Therapy except Reiki Master.

Reiki Touch Therapy was applied with Amanda augmenting her treatments. She came approximately twice a week, sometimes more, sometimes less, for about six months. Even though the treatments resulted in less pain for a short period afterwards, the repositioning of the bones in her feet perpetuated the pain to a degree she was no longer willing to tolerate. Amanda sought out the best orthopedic foot specialist available. This was no ordinary foot surgery. Amanda was to have seven procedures resulting in a full reconstruction of her foot.

Prior to her surgery I performed Reiki on her head for calmness, and on her foot for an hour. The operating arena was uncomfortable having me in with Amanda, so I did distance energy focusing from the waiting room.

The nurses were kind enough to come and tell me in which room Amanda would be so I walked to another floor to wait for her. She was mostly asleep but also aware that I was there. She pointed to her foot and to my hands, which I correctly interpreted as to begin Reiki on her foot.

This was about midafternoon. Around eight, Amanda's sweetheart, Bill, came in. Bill had also been trained in Reiki so he could offer support for Amanda as well as understand her condition. Even though Amanda would have liked for me to stay all night, I needed a break and Bill wanted some time with her.

The next morning I returned and spent the day performing Reiki Touch Therapy on Amanda's head and foot. The Reiki on her head provides understanding and promotes relaxation while the Reiki on her foot lessens the pain and hastens the healing process.

Amanda went home with a cast, braces, crutches and lots of medicines. Bill was a saint, helping her and just being with her during this trying time. Every day I administered Reiki for Amanda. Almost immediately she could get into a walking cast, then take it off altogether and with some surgery-friendly shoes, could ambulate around her house—now without pain. Her bones were now reconstructed so the muscles were re-routed to conform properly in place. The surgical scars are nonexistent and so far no scar tissue has been detected.

Amanda attends rehabilitation sessions when she feels like she needs them. However, her life is a total turnaround. Amanda has advanced from being an isolated invalid and in pain all the time to going out anytime she wants. She and Bill are always traveling on short and long trips. Amanda is now out of her second Saturn return. Her "understanding" has to do far more than just with her foot. Saturn's gift to her was more than a reconstruction of her foot. It was a reconstruction of her body, mind and spirit. She has become a more evolved and transformed individual with an enjoyment and acceptance of life.

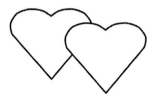

STRESS MANAGEMENT

It is a fact that life is busier than it used to be. Technology has created the planet as a "world village." There are no more mysteries to "going abroad" because everyone goes, or can go on the Internet. The world has been handed to us on a platter, not necessarily silver, but do we want it all? Our bodies, minds and spirits are taxed beyond degree. Illnesses are rampant, judgments are awry and it seems that it is all a big bucket of nuts and bolts.

We have certain ceremonies and rituals in my university-level Stress Management course. The students are graduating seniors, either going out into the business world or preparing for graduate school or sometimes both. I always arrive in the class a half hour or so before the students. This is to prepare the room for managing and reducing stress. The first thing I do is write a big "Welcome ☺" on the board. I use colored chalk and, as you noticed, put a smiley face or sometimes a heart, daisies or something sweet and fun after the word. If someone speaks to you with the word "welcome" it is a nice gesture. If there can be a visualization of a smiley face, a heart or a rainbow after that word, it takes on a connective energy form. Then the receiver truly feels welcome.

The next item written on the board is a quote, "Discipline Equals Freedom," by Krishnamurti. The word "welcome" and the quote, "discipline equals freedom," are on the board each and every class period so that is the first thing the students see. If one is disciplined in all ways, then freedom evolves, thus managing and reducing stress.

I bring a little scented candle in a pretty holder and have that lit before the students arrive. A portable compact disc player has soft, meditative music wafting through the room. The classroom door is closed during the class and as each student comes and goes. This provides a safety zone, a cocoon, if you will, and eliminates any noises from the hall. Next, all the papers required for the class have a certain place. A separate table is the designated assignment area.

The papers are divided into sections: those we need for the class that day, and those already graded and ready to give back to the students. There is a roll sheet, a stress measures sheet, and other papers pertinent to the class. The organization is in the same pattern each class, each week, for the duration of the semester. The students can depend on this, and it alleviates worry while creating and instilling a sense of order and repetition. It is a small and subtle idea but, over time, it works. Part of reducing and managing stress is this repetition, or practice, of certain techniques.

As the students file in, a definite notice of calm and peace is evident. In this class there are no loud voices; it is polite and honorable to be on time and to inform me ahead of time if any variation in the class will happen. There are no cell phones, palm pilots or laptop computers; almost no noise at all. The assignments have been set for the entire semester from the first day, so there are no surprises, and therefore, no anxiety as to what may or may not be required. This provides a peaceful and calming environment. Just as I am organized, calm and honorable with them, they know the same is expected of them. This educates them in responsibility and dependability.

Smiling, I cast a soft glance over the class to gain an internal register of their state. I note the set jaws, the tired eyes, slumped shoulders; all the burdens graduating seniors carry. They are allowed to chew gum or eat snacks during class and many times I bring this. Chewing gum is statistically proven to lower stress levels; it relaxes the jaw and prevents the clinching of teeth.

Sensing that a stage of equanimity has been attained, I take a deep breath and audibly let it out. I repeat that. We then proceed into our ceremonies and rituals. Ceremonies can change; rituals are set. The first ceremony is a four-step breathing exercise. We inhale on a three count, hold the breath on a three count; exhale on a three count, and hold that on a three count. This is repeated three times. This is a ceremony because the number counts may vary. I use the three count to teach the honoring of the body, mind and spirit. Many individuals count to seven or to ten, or some other number. My theory is to keep the number three and have longer inhalations or exhalations. Talk show host Larry King once asked Andrew Weil, MD, what was the simplest and most effective stress reducing measure, the answer was the breath.

Our next ceremony is the "Ah" breathing. We place our hands on our solar plexus and take a deep half breath; raising our hands to our chest we complete the deep breath and exhale with "ahhhhhhh." We repeat this action three times. The eyes may remain open or closed with these practices.

We do close our eyes for the "Om." We form our mouth into the shape of an "O"; take a very deep breath, and with half the exhalation sing O. Then we close our lips and complete the exhalation with Om. We also repeat this three times; for the body, mind and spirit.

A pharmaceutical company did a study stating that if the physiology is changed the emotions are affected in a positive manner. You may have heard psychologists suggest this to a depressed individual; to get up and move around, to generate some energy in the body, which will increase the endorphins in the brain and make the patient feel better. This next exercise is similar. It is called "Grinning." Each student makes eye contact with another student and begins to grin widely; from ear to ear. After the eye contact is made with one student, we move to another and then another, until all in the room have had eye contact and have been "grinned." By this time we are all giggling and laughing. We applaud each other after this, which also raises the energy level in the room.

We discuss cultural methodologies of reducing and managing stress. One is an Eastern philosophy regarding anger management. This philosophy is to understand, apologize and let go. Even though complete understanding may not be possible it is mature to apologize and our stress levels will be reduced when we let go. The Western approach to anger management can include mediation: two parties with opposing views and a mediator. Each party calmly states the facts; not emotions, to the mediator. The two parties know that each will have to make some compromise. After all facts are stated, and compromises are agreed upon, the mediator draws up a contract to which each party will adhere.

ASSESSMENT
Managing and Reducing Stress

1.   Methods in which I support myself in reducing and managing stress.

II. Methods in which I do not support myself in reducing and managing stress.

"STRESS TRIANGLE" AND OTHER AREAS
With gratitude to Lois Levy, MS, *Undress Your Stress*

PHYSICAL RELAXATION TECHNIQUES

Our muscles tighten to prepare us for the fight or flight response. Also, when our muscles shorten due to waste product build-up, tension and pain results.

- NECK ROLL
  Put your right ear to your right shoulder, keeping your left shoulder pulled down. Roll your head forward so your chin is on your chest. Now, put your left ear on your left shoulder, keeping your right shoulder pulled down. Do this, side to side several times. Now, roll your head to the front, as before, but continue on to the back and roll your head all the way around three times one direction, followed by three times in the opposite direction. Remember to deep breathe during this.

- SHOULDER SHRUG
  Draw a big circle with your shoulders. Right shoulder first, then the left shoulder. Rotate each one individually three times, then together three times backwards and forwards.

- STANDING MONKEY SWING
  Stand and allow your body to gently fall forward with hands and arms hanging down loosely. Begin to sway, side to side, and slowly observe your body swinging.

- PICKING FRUIT
  With one hand, reach up, as high as you can, and pretend you are picking an apple, peach or some kind of fruit from the tree. Stretch with your whole body as high as you can. Now, switch hands and repeat. Do three times.

~Seven Days of Affirmations ~

It is rewarding to smile! ☺

I enjoy giving and receiving love ☺

I am completely relaxed and at peace at all times ☺

I am great ☺ I am powerful ☺

I begin each day with excitement and energy ☻

Opportunities are headed my way now! ☺

Today is a wonder-filled day ☻

STRESS FACTORS

SEEKING RELIEF FROM STRESS BY
SMOKING, DRINKING, ALCOHOL, DRUGS, NOT
EXERCISING, OR EATING DIFFERENTLY WILL
CREATE SERIOUS HEALTH PROBLEMS ☹

DIFFERENT PEOPLE HANDLE STRESS IN
DIFFERENT WAYS. WHEN YOU FEEL
STRESSED JUST ASK YOURSELF IF IT IS
WORTH DYING FOR ☹

THERE IS NO SINGLE SOLUTION TO
HANDLING STRESS. CHOOSE THE STRESS
RELIEVERS WHICH SERVE YOU BEST ☺

☺ CONSIDER & CHOOSE FOR DAILY USE ☺

BREATHING EXERCISES	DAILY MEDITATION
BIOFEEDBACK	YOGA
KNOW YOUR STRESSORS	TAKE ACTION
MASSAGE	EXERCISE
NUTRITION	PRACTICE, PRACTICE
PROFESSIONAL HELP	SUPPORT SYSTEM

The Many Parts of Me

All of us are made up of many different parts, and special experiences help to form our personality. Each event, whether positive or negative, is just one piece of us.

Directions: On each puzzle piece write a different experience that was significant in your life. If you can recall, write how old you were when this experience happened. Some will be easy to remember and others may not. It may help to quickly review each year of your life. Example: "When I was six years old, my grandfather died." Later you may desire to journal your memories.

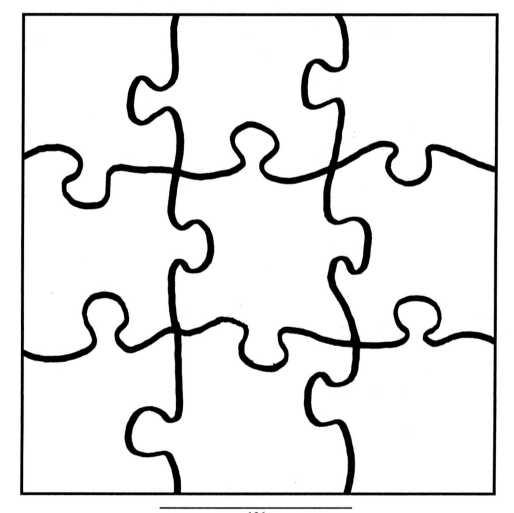

ESTABLISHING PRIORITIES/TIME MANAGEMENT/DAILY

Date: _____

What MUST be done TODAY!

1. _____

2. _____

3. _____

Affirmation: _____

What MUST be done but not necessarily TODAY!

1. _____

2. _____

3. _____

Affirmation: _____

What could be done at some other time and possibly ignored?

1. _____

2. _____

3. _____

Affirmation: _____

I AM GRATEFUL FOR: _____

_____

_____

_____

_____

_____

_____

ESTABLISHING PRIORITIES/TIME MANAGEMENT/MONTHLY

Date: _____

What MUST be done this MONTH!

1. _____

2. _____

3. _____

Affirmation: _____

What MUST be done but not necessarily this MONTH!

1. _____

2. _____

3. _____

Affirmation: _____

What could be done some other MONTH and possibly ignored!

1. _____

2. _____

3. _____

Affirmation: _____

I AM GRATEFUL FOR: _____

_____

_____

_____

_____

_____

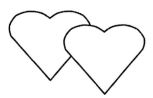

FINANCES

- Have a self or a family budget meeting once a month to be aware of extra or out-of-the-ordinary expenses that particular month. Example: school uniforms, braces, insurance payments, car maintenance, new clothes, other.
- Know where your money is and what it is doing at all times (in the bank, which investments, other).
- Keep a record of weekly and monthly spending; daily if you can.
- Review this record every three months, keep what you must have; delete the others.
- Pay your inspirational source 10% first.
- Pay yourself 10% second. Investments, real estate, savings account, etc.
- Have an accountant or a financial advisor. Banks have advisors for free. Most banks have a printed budget form and they will go over it with you.
- Reward yourself accordingly with the task or income produced from the task.
- Have one credit card that is also a debit card so the money is directly taken from your checking account.
- If you have a business, have a separate credit card for accurate records.
- HAVE NO OTHER CREDIT CARDS. They create illusions of wealth and

create true stress and anxiety.
- Read Suze Orman's books, listen to her tapes, watch her on TV, look at her website . . . suzeorman.com.
- Read Napoleon Hill's *Think and Grow Rich Action Pack* book. Do the actions. Write down your financial goals. Read them once a day.
- Buy a copy of *Success* magazine one month, *Money* magazine the next month, and one financial oriented magazine a month for six months. Decide which one suits you and subscribe to that one . . . only one.
- Buy what you need and do not buy what you do not need; exception is your reward gauged by your income derived from the task.
- Keep your checkbook in a place where you pay your bills and pay your bills once a month or twice at the most. Use your debit card instead of your checkbook for gas, groceries, medical, dental, school tuition and clothes. Your bank statement provides a printout for that.
- Have a list of what "miscellaneous" means in your budget.
- Keep "emergency" money separate from "miscellaneous" money.
- If possible, pay insurance, tuition and any other expenses annually.
- Decide an annual budget at the end of December and plan known expenses. This can include next year's Christmas budget, birthday parties and presents, and vacation expenses. Be aware of the age and condition of your home, your car, your physical self and that of your family's. Who will need dental work, eyeglasses, hearing aids, nursing home care? Some of these you actually know, and then when that time comes you have already written it down into the budget.
- "I cannot afford to live." Yes, you can. Make sacrifices; be willing to do that no matter how well educated or how old you are. Be willing to live beneath your means until you are out from under the money pressure. Learn to barter services.

Money

M oney is a subject that, of course, has no interest to anyone. In fact, I almost did not include it in this book. Just kidding. Actually, my next book is solely about money so this will be just a short chat with a few tidbits and perhaps one story.

Just as the protection chapter begins with the reason for being on the planet is to serve God and mankind, this chapter will also begin in this same theme. We do have a loving and generous Maker. Our Maker truly wants us to be comfortable and to have a reasonable enjoyment of life. I would venture to say, even though I have not read them all, that most scriptures have traditions about money and honoring the One from whom all blessings flow.

I grew up in the Deep South, in the Southern Baptist tradition, where tithing, or giving one-tenth of one's income to the church, is a given. It is a habit and the entire church budget depends on it. From the time I was born, any money given to me had one-tenth taken out to be given in the offering plate every Sunday. After I was old enough to receive an allowance it was understood, without question, that the first ten percent would be tithed. Even though I now disagree with the tradition of the Baptist definition, which is, if you do not tithe, you will go to hell, I still do believe and practice tithing. Why?

I believe that God created everything. This includes money. I believe that tithing money brings money back to the giver. There are rules about this, too, of course. The giving has to be with a good heart. The giving has to be with no thought of attachment to how the money will be used. In other words, the money is given freely, to be used however the receiver intends. I believe that God gives us one hundred percent of our money, with no strings attached, and only wants one tenth back. That is really a pretty sweet deal.

Some people say that they give God their time, instead of money. That is fine because God certainly does need everyone's time. And, when you give God your time, you are rewarded with more time. Think about it.

A few years back I was involved in a car accident that kept me bedridden for eight months and left me in braces, crutches and a wheelchair for several more months. I get paid when I work, so I did not get paid while I was flat on my back recovering. I had only worked three months that year, from January to March. The accident was the first week of April. At the end of the year, my

CPA informed me that my income was exactly, within about a thousand dollars, what the previous years income had been. No way. I called my business manager and he astutely said, "Don't you know Who your Source is?" That did not register with me.

Within two or three months after recovering from the car accident, I was mugged and beaten up, resulting in an eleven-month recovery period. I was not working again. At the end of the year, my CPA called to tell me that my income, for the third year in a row, was approximately the same. Again, I telephoned my business manager with this astounding announcement. He again asked me, "Don't you know Who your Source is?" I began to cry, not understanding at all. He told me that he knew that I always gave a minimum of ten percent to God. I agreed, but still did not get his point.

He told me that no matter how much or how little or how hard or how easy I worked, that as long as I honored my Source, then money would come in. I began to cry. I had a breakthrough, if you will, about my money. Yes, I had given the ten percent to God. It was the other ninety percent that I held onto for dear life. That money was mine, all mine, and nobody, not even God, could tell me what to do with the remaining ninety percent. As my business manager patiently listened he asked me how I felt now, with money coming in and I was not working at all. I told him, and I am telling you. All money is God's. Every penny. God gives us everything, including money, to manage for Her. When we properly, with honor and respect, with love and generosity, manage Her money, then we always have it. We are happier, more content, healthier, and have a stronger belief in a Higher Power who looks over us. Give to God. It works.

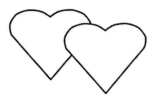

TRUTH
What is Truth?

Webster states that truth is to be valid, to be credible, to be believed. That truth is a state of being in accord with fact. That truth is avoiding distortion and is unadorned and naked.

Truth is truth no matter what we perceive it to be. When we tap into it and understand it we become it.

In the *Bible*, from the book of Proverbs, it is written, "that the lip of truth is established forever." In Psalms it states, "His truth endureth forever." In the book of John, from the New Testament, it says, "Ye shall know the truth and the truth shall set you free."

Truths are God's rules and regulations of what is.

Truth is all we have.

Disraeli says, "Time is precious, but truth is more precious than time."

The truth of the moment is that truth is constant change.

Krishnamurti, in his book, *Freedom From the Known*, tells this story: A great disciple went to God and demanded to be taught truth. God says, "My friend, it is such a hot day, please get me a glass of water." The disciple goes and knocks on the door of the first house he comes to and a beautiful lady answers. He falls in love with her, they marry and have several children. One day it begins to rain and rain, torrents of rain. The streets were flooded and houses were being washed away. The disciple runs to God and cries, "God, please, save us!" God asked, "Where is that glass of water I asked for?"

In *Darshan*, SYDA Foundation's publication, the June 1988 edition states, "Let your conduct be marked by right action, including study and teaching of the scriptures; by truthfulness in word, deed and thought; by self-denial and the practice of austerity; by poise and self-control; by performance of everyday duties of life with a cheerful heart and an unattached mind.

"Speak the truth, do your duty, do not neglect the study of the scriptures. Swerve not from the truth. Deviate not from the path of good. Revere greatness. Do only such actions as are blameless. Whatever you give to others give with love and reverence. Gifts must be given in abundance, with joy, humility and compassion.

"If at any time there is any doubt with regard to right conduct, follow the path of great souls, who are guileless, of good judgment, and devoted to truth. Thus conduct yourselves. This is the command of the scriptures."

The poet, Keats, says, "Truth is beauty, beauty is truth. That is all ye know on earth and all ye need to know."

Shakespeare said, "What is man, if his chief good is but to sleep and feed? He that made us has given us a Godlike capability that He did not expect to go unused. That Godlike capacity is the ability to perceive the higher will that runs through all of life. Ultimately, it is the capacity for knowing the truth of one's own being, the truth of the Self."

Again quoting from *Darshan*, "The words, law, righteousness, duty, religion and virtue all come under the meaning of truth." The Old Testament speaks of it as "God's law." The Greeks spoke of "noble excellence," the Chinese say, "correct order," The Romans use "virtue," in the east, Indians say, "dharma, or right action."

Socrates said, "That nothing evil can befall a good man, whether if life or in death. Upon truth everything is founded, therefore truth is called the highest good. Truth is so called on account of its capacity for sustaining the world."

Every human being who ever pondered the question of what is good, of what is right, comes in the end to the same conclusion: that there truly is a law, a force, an eternal thread of righteousness, which runs through all of life, with which all beings must align themselves if they are to be happy.

When we want the truth, we care—we have to give our whole attention to caring. That means we really seek to understand truth and we give our whole heart and mind to find it. Such a state of attention is total, and the totality of who you are is revealed in an instant!

Truth is Universal Law.

When Truth has a capital letter it is a noun.

We also look at truth as an adjective.

When we become truth, it is a verb; it goes into action.

The February 1988 issue of *Darshan* talks about truthfulness in its fullest sense: a commitment to truthful practice so complete that it will allow no gap between one's words and one's actions. In politics truth is regarded as naive. Truth is considered rude in social affairs, where white lies are expected; truth is considered unnecessary with the IRS and dangerous in personal relationships. We lie to protect ourselves from some real or imagined threat, out of laziness, or because we want to present ourselves as smarter or more courageous or more intelligent than we are.

Truthfulness is not practiced to make us better citizens but for the sake of stillness of the mind. Falsehood will immediately, in any form, throw us off center and out of alignment with the Self, which is of the nature of pure truth.

For many people, beginning to practice telling the simple truth can be an act of tremendous courage and discipline, one which reverses habits of a lifetime.

Mahatma Gandhi once pointed out that when a person has committed himself to telling the truth he also commits himself to being careful about everything he does. If one has sworn to speak the truth, one's actions have to be such that one is tempted never to lie about them.

A mother brought her son to a great teacher and asked for guidance. "Bring him back in two weeks," the teacher said. In two weeks the teacher told the boy to stop eating sugar. The mother, indignant, asked, "Why didn't you tell him that two weeks ago?" The great teacher replied, "First, I had to stop eating sugar myself."

Socrates used to tell his students, "We have to be what we want to seem."

The Yogic scriptures say that we do not know the truth or do not feel we can tell it then it is better to keep silent. On a level, truth is a matter of individual perception. Most agree that we have to judge the truthfulness of a statement by the inner attitude of the person making it. Baba Muktananda®, a great Siddha Meditation Master, said, "We must cultivate virtuous qualities."

Gurumayi Chidvilasananda®, the head of the Siddha Lineage and Muktananda's heir, states, "According to the Great Beings, speaking the truth means being honest with yourself. For that, you have to know who you are."

When we train ourselves to speak truthfully we also train ourselves to think before we speak. Truth is a delicate practice. A truth which causes harm should not be spoken or even thought! Gossip may be factual but certainly isn't beneficial.

Gurumayi® says, "To be able to see the truth we have to be able to see with God's eye, to see without the veils that ordinarily cloud our perception."

Practicing truth vigilantly and with our best understanding keeps us aligned with higher truth. If we say something we know to be untrue we create a separation within ourselves. When a person has become established in the truth, when words and thoughts and actions are in total alignment, then his words become infallible.

There is no way to pretend with God. God sees through us, but with unconditional love. In the mirror of God's gaze we see our own lacks, our tendencies to cover up some things and to display others. Then, we learn to see through God's eye, the eye of absolute love. With this we discover how we do not have to pretend. As we drop our pretenses we experience more deeply how truth sets us free.

In this writing we notice the words: eternal, always, forever, sustaining and endureth. These words have the quality of truth. Truth never stops; it is there always. We have to desire to know anything we want to know. We learn by trial and error and pain and pleasure what works for us. We try to escape; we try to sleep. Truth will always wake us up, sooner or later! We may say we had a rude awakening! That is when truth taps us on the shoulder and says, "This way, not that way."

We have had many lifetimes, everyone seeking for truth, for God, who is this Truth. We have experienced different planets, different cultures, different lifestyles, all growing toward God.

To be one with God is why we are here. We cannot escape our being or our creation in love. That is who we are. We must, with every breath, every thought, every action, seek and strive to attain this oneness with God, this Love, this All, this Truth.

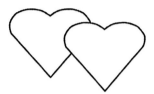

EXORCISMS

This would be the last thing I would ever want to do. Whenever, as a healer, any client would ask me about the subject, I would refer them to someone else. I wanted nothing to do with this work at all. Perhaps I had been influenced by the movies depicting the horrors of it, or perhaps my strict religious upbringing or being very afraid of "the devil." I truly knew nothing of the process and did not want to know anything.

In 1985 on a trip for a healing seminar, the teacher asked me how I was doing with the exorcism practices. I calmly, on the outside, said I knew nothing of it and did not practice it. Inside, I was quaking. She then proceeded to ask me how many people in the last six months had asked me to do this for them or for a family member. Taking a deep breath and letting it out very slowly, I answered that several had. She asked me what I did about it. I said that I referred them to a "ghostbuster" and weakly tried to make a joke about it. She told me that I should by now know that when someone repeatedly asks me to do something that it is an indication that I should do it. I protested loudly and, acting resentful, said that this was not the purpose of my trip, that it was for the other healing work.

She told me that I should know by now that we are never doing anything for the reason we think we are doing it and that one thing leads to another. While she was talking, I was wondering how in the world she knew that people had been asking me? After a few days, she convinced me that so many lost souls wanted bodies; and because of diseases, accidents, depression, abuses and other maladies, individuals are open to other entities coming in. These are usually not people who know protection methods or are very advanced in spirituality. This teacher also stated that most of the patients in mental institutions were there because of this entity invasion situation. I wanted to flee.

After a while I was convinced to at least listen to what the teacher had to say. The next time someone asked me to do some work of this sort on a family member I agreed to try.

The first thing was to completely protect myself. I would use everything available. Have a designated room. Protect the room in which the procedure would take place. Cover or remove mirrors. Close windows and draperies and close all doors into the selected room. Next, I would create a boundary in which the work would be performed. Virtually every tool I would need had to fit inside this boundary. Once I began the exorcism, both the subject and I could not leave the circle.

Now, what is "the circle"? The circle can be anything I decide will hold and maintain the generated power. For example, earlier in the book, flowers were mentioned as having great ability to absorb negative energies. The well-known Dr. Stanley Krippner gave a seminar about removing entities. He discussed a South American woman who was believed to be possessed. The Curandero, or shaman, took a bunch of flowers and, from head to toe, vigorously swatted the woman with the flowers. Afterwards she was no longer possessed. It is, of course, common knowledge that flowers raise the energies of a room or a space.

Salt is also good for protection. Crystals can be programmed to keep the energy in a specific area, too. Any pure silver is a very good protection. You give the power to whatever is used. You must believe that the circle contains the power to do what you need it to do. Love and gratitude are the primary components to empower anything. As the circle is being arranged, fill it with words, thoughts and actions of appreciation for their part in the success of the work. High energy or light energy is love energy.

Okay, back to the circle. The other items you may have in your circle could include a chair for the exorcism subject. This person must be in the chair and not leave for any reason whatsoever while the circle is being prepared and until the process is completely over. You may also have a chair for yourself. I prefer to sit on the floor. Include any power objects such as crystals, a Native American totem animal object, more flowers, holy water, which you prepared yourself, and your own good, sound mind. Your plan must be solid and intact. You must know exactly what you will do because the entity has a vested interest in staying in this person's body and will make every attempt to distract you. You and your subject must not have anything to ingest. Have no water, gum or food of any sort in your mouth. The process can take one, two or three hours, including the circle setup time.

Let us say that the circle is made of flowers. It must be unbroken, so overlay the stems or have an abundance of flower petals in an unbroken line. You can reinforce this with an unbroken ring of salt if you like. Have some supportive music playing; music which is calm and will assist you in concentration. Once you have protected yourself and have everything in place you may begin.

There is always a guardian angel at the subject's right shoulder. This guardian angel is for the entity which will be removed. There is an additional guardian angel at the subject's left shoulder. This is the subject's guardian angel. Sit directly in front of your subject. Do the protection around your subject as an added protection for you. Do not engage the entity with conversation and do not allow the entity to engage in conversation with you.

The entity will move around the body. This is to confuse you, to distract you, to hide from you, to make you think the work is done and for many other reasons. The entity may have occupied this subject's body and perhaps the soul for this lifetime and in many cases, several lifetimes. This subject's body is the entity's home and it will not want to leave. How do you accomplish this departure? With great love, perseverance and knowledge. Always have a teacher to instruct you in the many ways of these procedures. Do not take this small example as the one and only way to do this. Many details are not included in this brief illustration.

I sit on the floor about three or four feet away. I am not touching my subject. I turn my hands palms up and extend my arms toward the feet of my subject. My hands are strong and unbending. My fingers are straight out and rigid. Even though I may not be able to see the bottom or the soles of my subject's feet I send the energy there through my hands. I am working up toward the right shoulder where the guardian angel of the entity is waiting to receive it. Begin at the bottom of the feet and work up.

From there I slowly, very, very slowly, raise my hands through the foot. As I raise my hands, I am leaving a brilliant, golden light. A light that is too bright for an entity that is in the wrong body. A brilliant light in which the entity cannot hide.

I move up to the ankles, on up the calves, through the knees, the thighs, and so on. As I move my hands up, I am leaving the brilliant, golden light in the space I have cleared below my hands. I now enter the torso. This is generally where the entity is, around the base of the spine area, the stomach area and sometimes the breast area. The entity is fed by the desires of the subject, so sexual pleasure and food satisfaction are very attractive to the entity. Revitalize your focus because here is where the entity will dart around, or beg you not make it leave, or flatter you so you will weaken. You must be focused and have your goal firmly intact. Get it out of the subject's body and into the hands of its guardian angel.

Continue to raise your arms and hands. Go very slowly and advance upwards about an inch at a time, always leaving the blindingly brilliant, golden light in the spaces behind. Allow your vision to penetrate the subject's body. Go from front to back and side to side as you lift your hands. Be pro-active, alert and highly sensitive to the possibilities of the entity's mobility. With unwavering focus move on up, slowly, slowly. If you are diligent you will be successful. If you hear any noises, such as a dog barking, or a siren from a fire engine, or even something in the same room, rest assured the entity caused it. These are distractions. If you lose your focus you will have to begin all over. You do not ever want to begin all over. The entity will only strengthen in preparation for the next time.

As you arrive at the upper part of the torso bring your focus and your hands over to the left side of your subject. Use one hand to block and protect the area you have completed and use your other hand, palm down now, to move from the top of the subjects head down into the neck and over to the left shoulder. Now bring both your hands back together, palms up, and "corner" the entity in the right shoulder. The entity's guardian angel has his/her hands open and ready to receive this entity. Be aware that this is a frightened entity. This entity is being evicted from its home. This entity does not know its guardian angel and does not know that it is safe and will be taken to a proper place. This is where the entity may try to dive back into the body and hide. With the greatest of determination and persistence maintain your energy and focus. With great love, gently lift the entity out of the right shoulder and observe the guardian angel take it into his/her hands. The effulgent love of the angel will now fill the entity so it feels safe. Place your hands, palms down, over the right shoulder of your subject, again without actually touching the physical body.

If the guardian angel wishes it so, you may have the opportunity to witness the flight into other realms. The new home is spectacularly beautiful. Imagine beautiful architecture, lush green grass and trees, colorful and fragrant gardens, luxury of every sort and many other angels to welcome this entity. It is no longer homeless or lost. Here it will heal and grow strong enough to take birth and have a body all its own.

Now, address your client. Your client may or may not have closed their eyes during the process. Have the client now open them. Keep conversation to brief instructions. "Open your eyes. How do you feel? Slowly stand up." Be brief. Make an opening in the circle, large enough for your client to walk through. Have him/her go to another room. It is now all right for your client to have some water and to get comfortable. Ask your client to wait for you. No one else should be around.

You sweep, vacuum and totally clean up the flowers, each petal, all salt, and whatever else you used for your circle. If they can be flushed down the toilet then do so. Flush the toilet three times. If this is not possible due to bulk, they must be put into a sealed plastic bag and burned or emptied out into a running river or an ocean as soon as possible within twenty-four hours. As for any crystals or power objects you used for yourself, bury them a foot down in the ground for three days and nights. Bury them at night and dig them up at night. Completely cover them in a container of dry sea salt for the rest of the night. The next morning, wash them in room-temperature water with a mild soap. Place everything in the sunlight for the entire day. If the sun is not shining, use a bright, broad-spectrum lamp. Then, put them in the receptacles in which they are normally kept. They are now clean and can be used for other healing modalities.

Thorough cleaning of the designated room is imperative. I prefer a tile or wooden floor that can be mopped. After all the material is up and the floor is cleaned, I use an abundance of incense with the doors and windows remaining closed. I thank the incense for its work. After a few hours I will open the doors and windows.

The next instructions are very important for your client. Sometimes the experience leaves them with feelings of vulnerability or even abandonment or sadness. Something was in them for a long time and had become part of their vibrations. They may experience what some psychologists would label as an "empty nest" syndrome. When the client goes back home or to their hotel room they should immediately take a very long shower; not a bath. It is vital that all the vibrations of the procedure be showered off them. They should not have any other person in the room with them for the next twenty-four hours.

No engaging of conversation or intimacy is allowed. Room service or food delivery is okay, but keep conversation brief. Shower, eat and then rest, alone. They cannot let anyone touch them, especially in an intimate way, for this duration of time. The practitioner follows the same exact instructions.

As the client, after the twenty-four hours have passed, have a prearranged appointment with your practitioner, so you can touch base and begin to build new bridges for yourself. If your healer is trained in Reiki, have a minimum of four Reiki sessions, over the next four days, to provide balance and harmony for the new you.

As the shaman or healer, make yourself available to the client for at least a month. It will actually take six months or more for the client to be completely all right with the single energy now existing. Weekly psychotherapy from a knowledgeable and understanding psychologist, or regular contact with the practitioner, is best during this time. Keep good company, use substances that alter the psyche not at all or in moderation, listen to classical or meditative type music, learn to meditate and have a strong connection with a loving God.

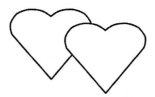

TAIWAN

Sometimes, as in this particular incident, the journey is a karmic one with lessons from the past bombarding you with an unexpected fierceness. When we sign up for our lessons in life it includes some tumultuous times. This is one of the painfully difficult lessons. This story is my opinion of my experience in Taiwan.

While staring out my high-rise window at a view that spanned many miles, I was wondering about other methods of wellness. I was about to have this wonder answered. Within a week of sitting in my comfortable home, I found myself in Taipei, Taiwan, enrolled in a healing course addressing the "chi." Seven American citizens had been invited to come and participate in an ongoing, multicountry activity. All the other countries were Asian. There was a dinner to welcome us and to exchange letters and gifts from respective mayors of our cities.

It did not take long for us to realize that we were objects of curiosity and we also detected some resentment, a protection of turf, so to speak. There were seven Americans and over a hundred Asians. None of the Americans spoke the language and indeed, there were many dialects. A translator explained that these other members of the class had also traveled long distances, but they had been studying for six months. They were wondering how we were going to learn all they had learned and become instructors in this form of healing in only three weeks. It was easy to understand their resentment. We did not know either.

In healing circles in the Orient, energy is a measure of one's worth and one's ability. The blend of the seven Americans included medical doctors, researchers with doctorate degrees, metaphysicians skilled in a variety of methods, and me, a Reiki Master. The translator walked to the other side of the room, mingled with the pointing fingers, and picked out a gentleman. The two approached me and the translator asked me to hold my arm and hand straight out. I obeyed this simple request. All the others there were closely observing the gentleman from across the room. With confidence and a smug smile, he moved his hand just above my arm and hand. I did not know what he was doing, but the translator did, and so did all his colleagues. His smug grin turned into awe.

He was surprised to discover that my energy impressed him and since he was impressed all the others were, too.

This was my first experience of "energy measurement" like this, so I was innocent of the process. However, I was not prepared for the stampede of the people on the other side of the room; all rushing to also touch my aura and to measure my energy. We were accepted into the group and the translator was happy and greatly relieved.

We left the next morning on one of many bus rides. There were several buses to accommodate about one hundred and fifty students and the instructor's assistants. The instructor was driven in a private car. We drove through very rural areas of Taiwan. For the most part the country was poor, but some of the buildings in the cities were magnificent. The Grand Hotel was a work of art and there were museums to rival the best in the world. Outside the museums and official buildings were soldiers who did not move, similar to the ones outside Buckingham Palace. It was almost as if they were wax statues. We watched them for a very long time and could detect no movement, not even breath.

As we arrived at one town, the home of the official Olympic training stadium, we were given a huge feast. The locals had the food prepared on the back of flatbed trucks, and it was brought in, course by course. The instructor sat at the head table with the country's dignitaries—governing members of agriculture, trade and commerce—along with other important officials.

Champagne flowed freely, followed by 7-Up. The food was mostly fish, rice and fruit. From my other Oriental travels I had come to not only expect but to enjoy having this menu three times a day. I was soon to appreciate this meal a lot more.

The entertainment came onto the stage. The performers were tiny five-year-old children. It was already late at night, but they were ready to demonstrate their art, Kung Fu. We certainly admired the talent and were amazed at the accomplishments of these babies. Upon closer observation we could not find a spark in the children's eyes. We could observe no enjoyment within the performers. They were like robots or puppets. We were stirred inside and uncomfortable. It was a premonition of things to come.

After this grand and delicious feast, we were escorted to our quarters. Even in the parking lot our hearts fell to a state where it had never before been. Looming up in front of us was a gray, cement structure, just straight walls about fifty feet in height. We could see into the entrance and noted the same gray cement bleacher-type seats. A part of us thought we were being shown this establishment as a sightseeing gesture, but the dead space inside of us knew better. A couple of the Americans staunchly refused to get out of the car. Others got out and eerily scanned the horizon for a taxi to take them to a hotel. Not to be. We were there as guests of the country and this was part of the package. I am sure the feeling of caged animals moved into our minds.

Inside was no better. The "rooms" were of solid concrete and had solid concrete bunks, with one sheet over it. We were given one paper cup. This would be to drink from, brush our teeth, and if necessary take our bath. We did not bathe for three weeks. There was a five gallon bottle of water in the room and it was used for everything. I will not describe the toilet facilities here. Imprisonment was on our minds and depression set in.

At five the next morning, with no one having slept a wink, one of the assistant instructors came yelling into our rooms. We gathered he was a human alarm clock. Alarm was appropriate. We were given some "uniforms" to wear; no changes included. After creatively attempting to brush our teeth and wash our face with the one paper cup, we were marched downstairs to the dining hall. It was all constructed of the same gray cement—walls, tables and benches. Our breakfast, as well as lunch and dinner, was being stirred over an outdoor-type gas flame. The two pots were huge enough to feed us all. In the pots were two items, soymilk and rice, one serving each in one bowl. We put the bowls to our mouths and drank the meal. Once a week, very proudly, we were served fish with this soymilk and rice. We will never forget the saving grace of our trip; one of our American ladies very casually reached into her purse and pulled out a jar of instant coffee. We just stared at her as she sprinkled this brown gold, with its fragrance wafting over to us all. Naturally, she shared it and we looked forward to that every morning.

After breakfast, the human alarm gathered us all, like cattle, onto the playing field. Nothing was play; nothing even approached a definition of frivolity. We marched, military fashion, onto the field. We Americans were allowed to have seven in our group; I think the language barrier was part of this. We marched in this fashion to every location for any and all reasons.

Our names were called and we had to respond with a straight-armed, military fist, and shout, very loudly, "Ho"! The exercises were interesting enough. It was very much like Tai Chi movements, but these were designed to bring balance and order to the internal organs and systems, with a vigorous and shaky movement. As part of the exercise we stood and stared about twelve feet ahead of us into the air; not at an object. Our tongue would be fixed on the roof of our mouths just behind our front teeth. Our knees were slightly bent and our arms hung down beside our hips. Somehow, just standing there in this posture, our bodies would begin to vibrate. The instructor, through the translator, said this was the body's innate "chi" or energy, moving through our bodies. Our hands would be the first to tremble and little, by little, the entire body would join in. As the body trembled we were instructed to do various movements or exercises, such as walking like a pelican, or other animal-named actions. This was Wai Don Gong.

The instructor paid a lot of attention to me. Even though there were at least a dozen groups for him to teach, he would come and stand in front of my group and watch me like a hawk. One of our group asked the translator why he was focusing on me so much. The translator answered that it was my energy and he could not stay away. The teachings were so precise and meticulous that it was very hard to remember. Even though the instructor was directly in front of us, he was speaking Chinese. I moved over close to the translator and tied a tiny tape recorder to my collar in order to get all the lessons.

One morning, either from exhaustion or the shock of the entire experience, I could not get out of my bunk. The other Americans were truly frightened because they had the concern that all would be punished if I stayed in the room. After they went down to breakfast I decided to put the tape recorder by my head, and with a low volume, began to play the instructions. Soon enough, the dreaded human alarm came racing into my room. There were no excuses to miss a class. These classes were twelve hours a day in the summer heat. Luckily I was flushed, had a temperature and must have appeared unwell. With a frown, I pointed to my head and my stomach, then to the tape recorder. I think he was convinced that I was indeed ill but I would be learning the lessons all day by my recorder. That was the only reprieve day.

Finally, the last day was arriving. We were holding our breaths because we felt that anything could jinx our departure. The translator came up to me and said that the instructor wanted my ring. I was wearing a gold ring which had been custom designed for me. I wore it all the time and was not about to give it up. That was the reason he wanted it; it had my energy in it. The translator convinced me that I had no choice in the matter, that I had to give it up. He also lamely attempted to inform me that this was a high honor. The translator assisted me with dressing and making me look as nice as possible, then led me out to an opening in a sparse garden. There were chairs in which the instructor and his assistants were sitting. The press was there, complete with photographers. I was guided to walk to the instructor, kneel and place my ring on one of his fingers. As I did this all the photographers surrounded us and bright lights were flashing everywhere. All the people were wildly clapping in approval. At that time a bird flew over and deposited a "gift" on my shoulder. The instructor and all the others just gasped. That was a gift and a message from heaven and I was surely blessed.

Another celebration dinner. We were all holding our breaths until we could touch ground in the States. More entertainment from young children and finally, a real meal. The instructor made a toast to all of us, but was looking at me while he spoke. I was invited to his table where he poured 7-Up into my glass and clinked his glass to mine and drank, as did I. Within ten minutes I was racing out the door with violent stomach cramps and nausea. Luckily there were medical doctors on our team, so I had someone with me. It was determined fairly quickly that I had been poisoned.

There was no hospital but two of the doctors took me to a hotel. I was shaking beyond belief and my eyes were rolling back into my head. I had no energy at all and had to be carried. We stayed in the hotel until it was time for all the buses to leave. The instructor was nowhere to be found. We all knew that I would not survive the bus ride, so a car was rented to drive the two doctors and me back to Taipei. We had to stop every few minutes on a normal five-hour drive. I was very ill.

We later found that it was lucky that there was no hospital. Because of the nature of the trip, the government would have kept me there. We checked into the Grand Hotel, a masterpiece built by General Chiang Kai-shek for his wife. After two days of hydrating me I was half carried onto the plane and on my way home. The doctors stated that I was in shock and was toxic due to poisoning, which we all later agreed to say was accidental.

It took at least six weeks of intense medical treatment before I was well. I lost part of my hair, had internal bleeding and lost a lot of weight. My lecture schedule was booked for me to make a trip to Chicago in another month. Cancellation seemed like a great idea, but I would be sharing the podium with some highly regarded, nationally known medical and academic doctors. So, I went. An older, genteel silver-haired lady came over to me in the afternoon of the first day. She took me by my hands and said, "Honey, what has happened to you?" I began to cry. She asked me where my room was and we proceeded to go there. We sat and had a cup of tea and I shared my story with her.

In addition to all the letters after her name, she was an accomplished clairvoyant. She did a guided meditation with me and saw that in a past life the Oriental instructor and I had been colleagues. We developed a formula that was going to make a great difference in pharmaceuticals. However, the instructor wanted all the glory so he had to get rid of me. He arranged a party, handed me a glass of wine and lifted his for a toast and we both drank our wine. Unbeknownst to me he had put ground up crystals into my wine. Not only would the crystals eventually cut up my internal organs and I would bleed to death, he also programmed the crystals to kill me. It worked and I died.

I related the incident in which I had to give my gold ring to him. She instantly knew that he was reconnecting with me in this lifetime to do his bidding, whatever that was. She asked me to draw a bath and to get into the tub. She came in, sat on the toilet lid, closed her eyes, and did another guided meditation that took all vibrations of the instructor out and away from me. She also took all my energy back from my ring and returned it to me. What the instructor ended up having was an empty piece of tin. We both had an image of a look of surprise on the instructor's face. I have had no other contact, in any way whatsoever from this instructor. The lady and I became close friends and shared in various lecture circuits for many years. I will forever be grateful to her.

Many people say that there is no proof of reincarnation. In my mind there is and this particular incident supported a lifetime centuries ago, and repeated, almost to the letter, again. I also believe that these reincarnation lessons can be healed. Proper guidance, of course, is mandatory.

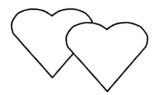

ART THERAPY
Art Therapy Methodologies

With Interviews from Jerry L. Fryrear, PhD and Irene E. Corbit, PhD.

Art therapy offers psychological or transitional space. This is the area, that is neither inside nor outside but bridges the subjective and objective reality. The burden is on the art therapist to provide and maintain a positive and supportive background or structure in order for his/her art therapy to proceed. When that is in place it is up to the therapist to match the appropriate art form to regenerate psychological space. The art therapist is, of course, focusing on images and symbols with the resulting expansion into the boundaries of objective reality. Cognitive/Behavioral Art therapy aids in recognizing truth. Thoughts produce images. In essence, the goal of Cognitive/Behavioral Art therapy would be to correct the thoughts and images. Such a correction must be based on behavioral evidence and logic in order to be perceived as truth.

Art therapy can offer a safe framework within which to investigate and experience the object world. The abstract but self-contained quality of the art mirrors the quality of the therapeutic relationship.

Interview with Jerry L. Fryrear, PhD

The following is an interview with Jerry L. Fryrear, PhD, addressing art therapy practices with preteens and teens. Dr. Fryrear was asked specifically how abused preteens and teenagers respond to art therapy.

Even though the age groups were varied with preteens and teens, it did not matter because abuse does not affect age. It can be like a character disorder, where a child is stuck at a certain age and not at the actual chronological age. The best way to work with this age is in a group format. The children could find common themes that supported them in not being alone in a situation.

One approach used in therapy was to begin with telling the child that he/she was an expert on child abuse. Since the child was abused the child knew more about it, and therefore was an expert for representing him or herself.

Next, I reasoned that life is not all bad. Even under the worst situations there are some good things. I tried to focus on the positive elements. If an abuse had occurred in a 24-hour period, then I would ask, what else happened in that same period? What happened that was good? I would ask the child to draw a picture about something good that was going on at about the same time.

The children felt punished by being taken away from their home and put into protective custody. They felt the abuser should be taken away, which frequently did happen, but the children were taken from their total environment. They were removed from their rooms, clothes, toys, school, teachers, other siblings and even pets. This was without exception. The system, which included the law, child protective services and the courts, felt like they were protecting the children. They were, in a great sense, but the children still felt punished and not only abused, but uprooted and moved to a strange place.

If a child has a safe harbor, a friend, a friend's parent, a grandparent, or a teacher, then these safe harbor individuals become natural therapists, who are not formally trained but provide the time to listen. Children will seek out these "natural therapists" to move from a discomfort space to a comfort space. Unfortunately, a lot of abusive parents will not allow children to visit friends or neighbors because they do not want the secret out. The parents also will not let other children come over and play. This happens in many ways, which serves to isolate the child.

One art project is in three parts. The first part is "Bad Things Happen," in which the child draws, paints or creates something that represents the abuse. Another segment is "It is Not All Bad," and the child creates the good or the positive things in their life. The art therapy part, which addresses the child's support system, is called "I Am Not Alone." This one uses an 8x11 or 11x14 sheet of white paper with amorphous outlines of twenty or more people. These outlines hint of males, females, adults, children, pets, perhaps super heroes, and gentle outlines, such as an angel. There is a dotted line figure in the middle where the child's photo is placed.

I then work with the child to find their true support system so they know who is really on their side. Many times the child will add something, perhaps a pet or an imaginary friend. I suggest that the child almost always has someone in the world to support and help him or her. Many times members of the therapy group are in there. We interact and ask if they do or do not feel supported by the group and why or why not.

The preteen and teen groups also discuss how being abused can lead to evil parenting. Some manifestations could be being completely self-sufficient so you don't need anybody, or becoming a bully and being so powerful no one will bother you, or becoming completely dependent on someone else so you never have to make any decisions. This can be translated into sayings such as, "If I'm loveable enough, no one will hurt me," or "If I am mean enough, no one will hurt me," or "If I stay away from everybody, then no one will hurt me."

A sequence of events is involved to engage the child's trust and willingness to participate in therapy. First, you get them to tell their own story, knowing the story is never complete due to memories being blocked or just not wanting to talk about it.

The psychotherapist and art therapist respond with, "I hear you say this is what happened, but I did not hear how this made you feel or what your reaction was." This technique is repeated until as much of the story is revealed as is possible. Then, the strengths are pointed out, which become apparent through talk therapy, art therapy or psychodrama.

Beware of psychotherapists who say things such as, "I am sure this happened, you just do not remember it." Or the opposite, "Did that really happen; are you sure; is that true?" This instills confusion and mistrust in the child. If it is true for the child, then it is true. This is the psychological truth and the therapist deals with that. One fact is that one out of every six women and one out of every ten men were sexually abused. Another fact is that the monster is usually right in your own house or very close.

Creativity is rapidly becoming the third therapeutic principle, with talk therapy first and talk-action therapy, psychodrama, being second. Crafts used to be the art modality but pain can be expressed in combinations of creative methods, such as drawing, painting, clay models and photographs. Dreams can be expressed artistically and impactfully.

Children think and talk in metaphors, so metaphors can be used in art therapy versus linear or logical therapy. Abstract symbols can indicate a change. One child drew a picture of his family in an airplane, except the child was outside the plane, hanging on to the tail of the plane. After several art therapy sessions the whole family was inside the plane. One girl drew herself with no hands, later drew her hands being behind her back, then later was handing, with both hands, a bunch of flowers to a friend.

Instilling hope in the abused child is crucial. Point out how far the individual has come and note all the achievements and accomplishments. Build on the strengths and successes. The abuse will always be there, but you can be a functioning person in spite of what happened to you. Every time you talk about it and work with it, the memories get easier to deal with. Don't ever let the memories run your life and keep you from being in charge. Visual journaling can give you a record of your changes as to where you were and where you are now.

Interview with Irene E. Corbit, PhD

When a child is painting or using crayons and the end result is one color, usually gray, brown or black, what does this mean? This usually indicates some chaos in a child's life. While noting and addressing the chaos and reasons for that with the child's primary caregivers, the child is guided to explore a different way. This is to ask the child what his or her favorite color is and to say that today we are going to work with one color, your very favorite color! The next time an additional color can be added and the child can work with two colors. If the child is confused or frustrated by this then teaching the child to mix and blend colors can be a diversionary tactic. Teach the child that blue and yellow make green and that combining red and blue will create purple, and experiment with others, one session at a time.

If anyone would be disinclined to seek therapy, for example, due to financial reasons or social pressure, what measures can be used to work out their current problems caused by childhood memories? Dr. Corbit suggests seeking out women's support groups or a close friend or confidant, a former teacher or the minister to aid in processing these memories. Read everything available on the particular abuse using a self-help modality. Take notes and begin affirmations to change your life.

If a client feels that they are a "walking mirror" and thinks that everyone around them can see their pain and former victimization, but cannot seem to pull out of this, what can be done? Dr. Corbit states that she would use the Adlerian approach of encouragement and support. Perhaps saying, "I know this is painful for you and has been a struggle for many years. Other women have also endured this and have overcome it. These memories will be hurtful, but we will work together and get you through this." Dr. Corbit describes a case study utilizing the Malaysian Senoi Dream Work.

Case Study Utilizing the Malaysian Senoi Dream Work

A mother and father, who are currently separated and planning to divorce, bring their child into treatment because of major changes in their child's behavior, which include poor grades in school, isolation from friends and nightmares. In what manner would you treat the situation? Describe your treatment plan for the child.

Treatment of the situation. First, obtain signed consent and confidentiality forms, which protect all parties. Meet with one or both parents, singly or together, with and without the child. Incorporate, if possible, marriage and family therapy communication with the parent(s)' therapists.

Have all pertinent factual information from parents, previous therapists, doctors, relatives, friends and anyone legally and ethically able to provide this. Have parent(s) in the therapy sessions but they must be silent and not intrusive. In order to give the parent "something to do," I could have them model my behavior by observing me and even give them notebooks to write down ideas in. This would empower and not alienate the parent.

Treatment plan for the child. Address the child as an adult. It is important to tell the child as much of the truth as clearly as possible because their imagination will fill in the spaces with fearful and false information and then act on it. Also, the artwork will change from chaotic to organized. (*Fryrear, Corbit, 1992*)

With a divorce situation and expected separation anxiety, the establishment of trust is vital. I would use positive reinforcement and behavioral modification and praise the child at every given opportunity. This will build self-confidence and self-awareness, which will support the child, regardless of what is going on in his/her life.

A simplified version of the Malaysian Senoi dream work would be very therapeutic for the child. The child could draw the nightmare or use photography to put himself/herself into the bad dream. The child could relate the nightmare while he/she does his artwork. Next, the child is asked to find a strong force or ally to take back into the nightmare. Anything that the child feels would protect him/her. Most importantly, the child feels totally safe before reentering the nightmare. They then ask the nightmare figure "how may I help you?" Then listen for an answer. Therein follows a gift exchange where the nightmare figure can change form or behavior to something positive. This act brings about inner harmony for the child who then transfers it to an art modality. A photo of the child with a strong, confident pose, possibly making him or herself a hero or heroine can provide for supportive and strengthening feedback.

Sean McNiff, PhD, suggests that the psyche expresses itself in a variety of forms and by providing a multimodal arts approach; the client is allowed multiple avenues for change and personal growth. Visual transitions therapy represents an advance in art therapy and has three basic components. One, the visual art therapy, two, the multimodal format which blends art, photography, movement, video and group or private psychotherapy, and three, is the built-in provision for metaphoric change. *(Fryrear and Corbit, 1992)*

Personal growth is a turning point, consciously and subconsciously. If a client is choosing personal growth it falls upon the therapist to be responsible and offer choices. Menard Boss emphasized that guilt occurs when choices are made; and in his book, *Man's Search for Himself*, Rollo May wrote about the anxiety and loneliness that confronts individuals in a modern society.

Power of Creative Process

Edith Kramer emphasized that the creative process has integrative and healing powers and when the child cannot verbalize the problem, talking is not required. Children should be offered a variety of media, particularly, according to Wadeson, "fact media" or media easily manipulated.

Children often feel quite comfortable with art media and can find a way to make themselves "heard," particularly in a family where it would not be possible for ordinary interactions. Also helpful to children of divorce and those faced with "fluid families" would be to have the parents, stepparents, girl/boyfriends, brothers, sisters (natural and step), to participate in multiple family art therapy.

Bruce D. Perry, MD, discovered that children who have experienced trauma will have smaller brains, and that the brain will not develop normally. He maintains that creative arts will aid in healing and balancing the child's physical body and brain, which will support the overall healing. Dr. Perry especially addresses the neurodevelopmental rationale for sequential enrichment, stating that to encourage abstract thought and to engage the cortical brain, use storytelling, drama, art therapy, writing and music. Also, to connect and involve the limbic brain and to facilitate emotion regulation, utilize dance, play therapy, art therapy, and nature discovery. Additionally, to engage the midbrain, which incorporates with somato-sensory integration, the techniques of touch therapies, such as Reiki Touch, along with music making and motion. The brainstem is also engaged through touch therapies, such as massage and pressure point therapy.

Bruce D. Perry, MD, formerly Chief of Psychiatry and Senior Fellow, CIVITAS Initiative, at Texas Children's Hospital in Houston, Texas.

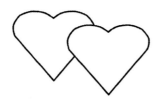

CHILD ABUSE
Celia and Nancy

One evening, around nine, a call came in from Texas Children's Hospital. The individual apologized for the late hour and asked if I was the author of the book, *Reiki Touch*. After I acknowledged that I was, she asked if I thought Reiki Touch Therapy would be a positive factor in healthcare for severely maltreated children age one to six years.

My response was that I believed that this modality helped all conditions, after which she invited me to come and speak to the physicians and staff about Reiki. She also asked me to bring my book, which she thought would validate my work. I was happy to do this and also wondered what this was all about.

The meeting consisted of other alternative healthcare practitioners, all presenting methodologies believed to aid these targeted children. The doctor in charge of this meeting was Bruce D. Perry, Chief of Staff of Psychiatry and Neurology there. He was a young man with credentials longer than can be written here. After hearing the presentations and meeting with each of us one-on-one afterwards, we all left. He was gracious and very interested in finding new and different ways to reach these catatonic and permanently damaged children.

A week or so passed and I was again invited to come to Texas Children's

Hospital to further discuss this program. Two little girls, now in foster care, would be evaluated that day and I was to observe them and consider being part of the program. There is no way any individual can be prepared for working with severely maltreated children. One would have to be a living heart donor to not be drawn in and deeply affected.

These two little girls, age nine months and eighteen months were barely functioning. Nancy, the nine-month-old was a "shaken" baby and had frequent convulsions. Her development was delayed by many factors.

Celia, the eighteen-month-old, had been thrown across a room, which resulted in a dented skull. Both were frequently shut up in dresser drawers and given liquor in baby bottles to keep them quiet. The birth mother had trouble getting them to eat solid food so would push the food down their throats with her fingers. This naturally set off the gag reflex so the infants would regurgitate the food. In frustration and lack of maturity the mother would injure the children.

Nancy had delayed motor development and would just sit in anyone's lap and stare. Celia, the oldest, was catatonic. She also stared, but with a terrified, wide-open-eyed look. She was rigid and rubbed her thumb and forefingers together to the extent of reaching the bone. She could and would cry as long as seven hours without ceasing.

Two other little boys were there that day. The parents had been on a drug binge and had placed both the one- and two-year-old in one crib for about three days. There was no food, no water and no change of diapers. The neighbors finally tired of hearing the baby's screams and called the police.

Rats had gotten into the crib and had chewed off the ear lobes, tips of noses and fingertips of these children. Child Services provided foster care for the boys. The parents were jailed for two days.

I was taken into a closed circuit video room. Here I could observe the children's evaluations by the doctors. The families were separated and I chose to observe the girls. I could both hear and see as the doctors, psychologists, foster mother and children sat on the floor. I saw the healthcare staff offer toys, crayons and books to the nonresponsive girls. After a half hour, Dr. Perry came into the video room, asked how I was with all this and did I think I could keep my composure in the room with the children. I wanted to flee, but nodded that I was ready to follow him into the room. Whenever anyone walked in or out of the room, or even adjusted their posture to reach for a toy, the children would be traumatized.

I happened to have worn a Disney decorated shirt, bright red with Mickey Mouse and Minnie Mouse on the front. This was safe clothing to the children. As I entered the room the children sat in the foster mother's lap and basically "married" the mother's body. Dr. Perry had cautioned me against making eye contact with the children, so I talked to the personnel while glancing, now and then, at the little girls. I had the idea that I would draw attention to the Disney characters on my shirt so I began to "talk" to Mickey Mouse and Minnie Mouse. This drew the attention of Celia and she leaned forward and touched the shirt. This was astounding to the healthcare professionals in the room. I used a breathing technique, an element of neurolinguistic programming, and matched my breathing pattern to hers.

As Celia continued to lean over I placed my hand, palm facing, near her back. I did not touch her. However, just that overt motion on my part caused her to quickly press her body into her mother's chest. My hand was in between, so now I was giving her Reiki. She did not notice and I endeavored to keep her attention on my shirt with my free hand. After a while the generated warmth of the Reiki raised her curiosity and Celia leaned forward and looked around at my hand. Slowly I brought my hand back to my lap. She was okay and she felt safe.

That was the end of that day's session. I was in a state of care and concern, not only for the children, but for myself, too. Could I handle this? I was willing to try. There were staff meetings twice a week for about six or seven hours each Tuesday and Thursday. At these meetings, horror stories in the form of medical reports would be presented. There were about ten staffers present and each one had two or more reports. One was a two-year-old boy whose father had been murdered in front of him. The toddler was left alone with the dead parent until the other parent picked him up after two days. There was a six-year-old girl who had been in twenty foster homes. In her natural parent home, and in all the foster homes, she had been raped by any and all male members in the families. She was put on heavy drugs to manage her mental state. The other reports were as serious or more serious.

I saw Celia and Nancy each Monday for two or more hours. Each time I would observe through the closed circuit video before I went in. This provided me with information as to their state that day. It was different each time. Due to the laws, the children had visitations with the birth parent. Each visit with the birth parent would send the children back to convulsions and seven-hour screams. The law was the law and also the birth parent was pregnant again. Each child had a different father. There were thirty-two adults in one house and the furniture consisted of upside down plastic milk cases.

I made a habit of wearing Disney motif shirts for each visit. It was something the girls could look at and not be afraid. After a few weeks of creative Reiki touching, the girls would look at me. I still avoided their eyes because of the obvious pain deep inside them. One week we were all astounded when Celia, the oldest, got up out of her foster mother's lap and walked across the room to get a toy. Progress was slowly happening.

Working here was probably the most difficult task I had ever encountered. The psychiatric unit was on the seventh floor. When I completed my work I would get on the elevator, walk through the lobby, into the parking garage and get into my car. Before I could put the key into the ignition I would surrender to uncontrollable sobs. I would cry without ceasing for a while. After that, in somewhat of a stupor, I would drive to the ice cream store and stuff ice cream, without tasting a bite, into my mouth. When I got home I would be nauseous and throw it up. This became a habit each time I left these children.

Once, on a regular check-up visit with my general practitioner, I happened to mention this assignment and my reaction to it. She was astonished and exclaimed that I was bingeing and purging. No way! However, she was correct. Even without being conscious of it I was acting out an eating disorder. Further, I began to cry at night, waking up and not being able to go back to sleep. One night as I was crying, I wandered to the sofa and looked out the window. My high-rise view was very pretty and especially soothing at night. As I sobbed, I felt I had a message from God. The message was for me to stay in my area of expertise and to only handle my piece of the pie. There were hundreds of children in this program, and I was hearing about all of them at the meetings, plus doing my own therapy with my assigned children. I stopped going to the meetings.

As more time passed I was able to hold Celia and Nancy in my lap and read a book to them. One hand was always doing Reiki Touch Therapy. Sometimes the older girl would begin to cry. We all dreaded that because once it started it did not stop. The plan was to entertain and distract her to encourage her to stop crying. I thought a lot about this. After a while I came to the realization that she had too many tears inside and they had to come out.

I told the healthcare professionals that I wanted to try something different; to allow her to cry as I performed Reiki on her. Thereafter, when Celia began to cry, I would pick her up. She was so tiny from being starved; it was like holding a rag doll over my shoulder. They did not know how I was going to endure all that crying. Neither did I. I held her as I walked out of the office, up and down the halls, the stairs, from room to room and from floor to floor. I had a little sing-song ditty, "Cry, cry, cry away. Cry, cry, it's okay." I would croon this to her the whole time. She was never too heavy. After many, many occasions of this behavior, she would cry for shorter and shorter periods, then go sound asleep on my shoulder.

I worked with these two children, as well as a few added ones, for several years. After the hospital program ended, they became my private clients. I became a family member, so to speak, attending birthday parties and special dinners. Most of the children have now been adopted into normal homes and are in regular school. They are happy, adjusted and we have a special bonding from the Reiki. Dr. Perry is a world-renowned physician with special interests for children. His program was considered too avante garde for Texas and the funding was discontinued. Dr. Perry is regularly featured on national television and magazines. We are very lucky to have someone of his caliber know and care for these special-needs children. Thank you, Dr. Perry.

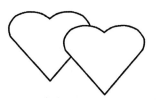

REGRESSION
Patti

atti was an adult incest survivor who had a call one evening from her father. She had not been in touch with him in about ten years and that was at her mother's funeral. He asked to come over and have a prayer service for the express intent of Patti forgiving him. This action was weighing heavily on his soul and he wanted to be able to peacefully face his Maker. In his mind, having Patti forgive him was a key element.

He said that other family members and friends also wanted to come to have a prayer circle, to pray "over her" so she would do this for him.

Patti was too taken aback to respond, so she asked him to call back the next day. Patti also noted that she felt thrown back into a submissive, childlike state and was quietly responding with "yes sir, no sir, please sir." She felt helpless and hopeless.

Even though it was after nine at night, Patti called a psychotherapist who knew of her background. Patti asked what she should do. The psychotherapist, a very wise and conscious woman, instructed Patti on several points.

Make a decision with the knowledge that you can change your mind even as the doorbell rings. You can just walk out the back door and hop into your car and drive away and never see his face. You decide who, if anyone, you want in your home. You decide how many people can come and for how long. Write a script of exactly what you want to say and do not change it. Plan ahead where each individual will sit. Do not serve coffee, tea, cake or water. This is not a social visit. Have a tape recorder hidden under the chair where your father will sit. As the doorbell rings, turn it on. Have a hidden video camera placed where it will be focused on your father and, like the tape recorder, turn it on when the doorbell rings. Do not touch him nor allow him to touch you; exercise the same behavior with the others. Sit in front of your father. You begin, carry out and end the conversation. You stay in charge the entire time.

Patti wrestled with the decision during the night. There was no sleep. By morning she had decided that her father could come and his sister and his sister's friend. No one else. Her father had wanted a total of seven or eight people but she said not this time. Around four that afternoon the doorbell rang. Patti had set the stage, the script was written and the recorders turned on. With her stomach in her throat, she opened the door. As she opened it, she moved behind it so he could not hug or touch her. She motioned for the three of them to come in. They had their *Bibles* clutched to their chests and had righteous indignation on their faces.

Three chairs were placed in a row with Patti's chair facing them. She instructed the two women that this was a meeting she had granted to her father; this was to be between her and her father. Further, they were not to talk unless invited to do so. This was clearly not part of the plan but Patti's father calmed them.

Patti began the meeting by asking her father at what age had the molestation begun. He was surprised at the tone of the visit. The women said, "We just came to pray!" Patti's father answered the question and many others that followed. The women were extremely disconcerted and interrupted several times to inform him that he did not have to answer that. He did answer all questions. He also attempted to invite Patti back into the family and have things "like they used to be." It was clear to Patti that he was not clear on the concept of how things were and now are.

There was no prayer circle, no *Bibles* opened and the meeting ended in less than a half hour. Patti informed him that forgiveness was for God and he should go there to ask for it, not to her.

After they left, Patti called the psychotherapist, who was waiting for the call. Patti felt confident that she had handled the process with maturity and expertise; she thanked the therapist and said she was just fine. The psychotherapist was very pleased that everything went so smoothly.

That evening Patti was not hungry for dinner, but did not think anything of that. She also wanted to watch some childlike cartoons but also felt that was natural due to the stressful afternoon. Later, Patti had trouble falling to sleep. When she did, dreadful nightmares, flashbacks and physical feelings of her father on top of her, left her gasping for air and feeling suffocated. She tossed and turned all night. There was no rest.

The next morning Patti awakened and as she sat on the side of her bed she was surprised that her feet could touch the floor. She got up, walked to the bathroom and looked around for the stool with which she used to stand on to brush her teeth. Somehow, she was able to reach the sink without it. She went downstairs and had a Mickey Mouse pancake with way too much syrup. She spilled the orange juice. Breakfast was just like she'd always had in first grade. Bacon, eggs and coffee did not occur to her. She looked everywhere in her closet for the red and white gingham dress with the white organdy pinafore, and somehow thought she found it and put it on. In her mind her mother braided her hair in French braids and put ribbons in to match her dress. She looked perfect. Patti always had to look and act just perfectly.

It was a school day so she made a peanut butter sandwich to take for lunch. Patti climbed into her car, wondering how a six-year-old could drive or even reach the foot pedals for that matter. She reached school and went to her classroom. She acted exactly like a six-year-old. She was fidgety, had a short attention span and kept wondering when this teacher was going to hand out crayons, and more important, just when was recess? In reality the class was in graduate school and was three hours long. Patti's regression back to age six could not manage that kind of time frame, so she got up and left. For the next three days, Patti lived as a six-year-old, sometimes there was a brief intervention wondering how she could do things a grownup could.

On Wednesday Patti had her promised appointment with the psychotherapist. She happened to notice it on a calendar but did not recall just why she had this appointment. She managed to find the building and sat in the reception room awaiting her appointment. She did a couple of exercises in the children's magazine, *Highlights*, while she waited. As the psychotherapist walked out to get her she jumped up and skipped into the therapist's office. Once in the office, Patti leapt onto the sofa, sat cross-legged and looked at the therapist in a "why am I here" look.

The psychotherapist rapidly realized that a six-year-old child, in an adult body, had skipped into her office. She began asking what Patti had been doing.

Patti stated, in a spontaneous, childlike manner, that her daddy had come to see her and she did not like that. The psychotherapist asked about the visit and received convoluted and scattered answers. After hearing Patti's story, the psychotherapist suggested a game. "Oh, goody," Patti exclaimed, "I like games."

The psychotherapist, using a skillful meditative process, led Patti from an even earlier age, through the current exhibited age six, and further into adulthood. The psychotherapist, chronologically, had Patti recall birthday parties, siblings, addresses, school friend's names, teacher's names, Patti's wedding date and husband's name, and many other reality-based facts. She took a great deal of time and patience with this process.

Patti finished this "game" and left. The psychotherapist called Patti two or three times a day just to chat, always speaking in present time to the adult. Patti was in the in-between stage of coming back into her real-time self. It took about two weeks and additional progression therapy to bring her back to her adult consciousness. It took several months to recover from the shock of the experience. Patti later said the Reiki Touch Therapy was a safe vehicle to bring balance and harmony during this searching-for-herself phase.

This experience for Patti was invaluable in countless ways. One, it revealed how strong her mind was. It demonstrated how the mind, body and spirit can be in another, yet familiar, form and still function. She understood that she went somewhere from which she might not have returned. Both Patti and her therapist grasped a greater understanding of how one could perform in more than one age and experience at the same time.

Many times, if one is thrown back into a previous age and cohort experience, it is impossible to return. The mind feels safe at the chosen regressed age and can comfortably build a life around that. This regressed age can affect the individual for the rest of her life. Patti is fortunate that she did come out of this. She has complete memory recall now of her father's visit. She gave the tapes to some authorities in the event anyone needs to know and have proof of his adverse behavior with his daughter. Amazingly, Patti has not renounced her father. She believes he has a mental imbalance and has, for her own peace of mind, forgiven him.

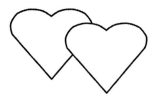

DOMESTIC VIOLENCE
Robby and Alex

I am a certified professional mediator. The mediation training included family law and domestic violence. The instructors included child psychologists, individuals who worked with child advocacy groups and protective services, along with attorneys and judges who had the legal responsibilities. One theme among all the teachers was that the children in domestic abuse situations developed severe illnesses, some life threatening. And, when records were followed throughout the late teens, apparent suicidal tendencies and chronic illness were observed.

In my holistic practice, there have been two young men who came from abusive homes. The situation in both homes was a case of the father abusing the mother. The mother carried the son in her womb for nine months, gave birth to the son and was, in every way, his mother.

The fathers in these examples verbally and emotionally ridiculed, minimized, diminished and in some instances, physically abused the mother. The son, wanting to love and adore his mother, was caught.

If he was to grow up and be a man, was this the role model from which he must learn? The son was torn, was given mixed messages. His heart could not open to trust his mother and his maturation and understanding of women was destroyed. He possibly thought this was being strong and manly, but his body did not agree, so there was always conflict, resulting in illness.

Robby was from an accomplished, socially proper family. He was well educated, a skilled polo player and an articulate speaker. Friends touted him for a future politician because of his ability to move in the "good ol' boys" circle. His ease with women was nonexistent and he only had sarcastic and negative views of women. The fact was that this side of him had never properly developed. As he matured, this void, this lack of appreciating and understanding the opposite sex threw him into a severe depression and he took his life. Afterwards, while counseling with family members, the history of what led to his suicide was revealed. The parents denied any part of the responsibility for this, but the siblings disagreed and supported the theories that led to the end of Robby's brief life.

The second young man, Alex, came from a family of academicians. Both parents had doctorates in complex scientific fields. The father was in constant competition with the mother as they worked for different universities. The mother, who worked diligently all day at her job, would come home and cook, clean, iron and very late at night, prepare for her work the next day.

Some say that guilty people become desperate people. Perhaps this is what occurred in this family. No matter how hard the mother tried to have the meals on time, the shirts ironed to perfection it was never good enough for the husband. The son could not thank the mother for a meal or for his room being cleaned. The father did not allow him to make up his own bed because that was woman's work. This woman also mowed the yard, kept the garden and even did the handyman repairs around the house.

When something was not done to the father's liking he would punch the mother, starting lightly on her arms or shoulders. He would laugh as if he was playing or making a joke. When the son was young he thought this was funny and not only laughed but would jump up and join in the "fun" of punching the mother. She did not want the son to know that she was in pain and would later be bruised, so she managed to laugh.

The husband would take the laughter as an attack at him, so he would escalate his behavior into punches in the stomach, across the back and places on her body that would be covered by clothes at work.

Alex grew up in this adverse surrounding and his attitude toward women was immature and undeveloped. He would not go to school dances or date. When his classmates could convince him to go, his behavior mirrored his dad's behavior with his mother. The girls soon did not want to date him and his reputation was in disrepair. His teachers viewed him as a troubled young man with some kind of imbalance that would reveal itself later. Yes, that is what happened. However, the imbalance was an illness, a life threatening and catastrophic illness, cancer.

The mother quickly called me and asked me to treat her son. I knew the family and of course wanted to help. I had to keep these treatments a secret from the dad because the ramifications at home would be too severe. The mother brought the son over each evening for Reiki Touch Therapy treatments. Sometimes she would stay and sometimes she would leave and come back to pick up Alex. When she stayed, I observed her sitting quietly and just imbibing the peaceful atmosphere in my office. A scented candle was always lit, soft music was playing, the lights were dim and there was a beautiful view of downtown.

The times she left, I noticed Alex taking a sigh of relief. He had already begun his traditional treatments of chemotherapy and radiation, so he was nauseated and disoriented. This was his time to talk. It was as if he had never, in his lifetime, had his time to talk. He would talk incessantly, almost afraid that I might say something and interrupt, which I did not. It was as if a dam of suppressed energy, saved for just over twenty years, could now let go. He spoke of his dad hitting his mother, of her trying so hard to please him, of hearing his bedroom demands and her begging him to stop hurting her, of never having a moment's peace in his own home. He said he did not plan on living to endure that atmosphere or to carry those learned behaviors into a relationship of his own.

As is my habit with anyone who has a diagnosed terminal disease, I encourage them to talk about their dreams, their vision, their future plans.

When they have none and get really confused with these questions, I can usually predict that they will not stay here. Alex had some plans, some hopes, some dreams. But, they were limited, short term, like passing a quiz in a class or seeing a new movie or going to the beach. I listened and gently suggested something further into the future, graduation, a new car, a European trip, all of which would require a lot of planning and time. He could not stretch that far.

Even with all the treatments of holistic and traditional medicine, Alex was, on some level, rapidly making a decision to leave this plane of existence. He had to move back into the home and was dependent on his quarreling parents to provide for his healthcare and regime. It was just too much for him. He could see no hope for a productive and peaceful life for himself. After about six months he passed away. The parents, to this day, are unaware of anything they did to contribute to this. The consciousness of their behavior affecting him at all, much less to the degree of causing an illness that would take his life was and is nonexistent.

Parents take heed that children must have love, safety and respect for all in their surroundings. Children must have a nurturing environment in order to survive, be healthy and to perpetuate that positive behavior as they grow and mature into adulthood. If adult abuse is being noted in mediation, child protective services, with lawyers and judges, then make changes. Alter your life to love and respect your spouse and give your children proper role models. It can mean their life.

PARALYSIS
Suzanne

After being in real estate and the corporate world of attorneys, business-men and business women, the world of healing as a business was a learning curve of great magnitude. Attending metaphysical workshops as an avocation and chalking it up to curiosity, I was all of a sudden brought to a screeching halt in my body, mind and spirit. Had I been training for something all these years?

About a week after the first level of Reiki training a medical doctor invited me to lunch. He had been in the same Reiki class and noted, according to him, my seriousness about the subject and my compassion with the other students. He commented that two doctors were leaving his medical center that would make two treatment rooms available. He had a desire to offer a wider range of healing modalities to his patients. He also had residents and interns doing rotations each month and wanted to educate them in holistic medicine methodologies. He invited me to join his staff and have a Reiki practice in his medical center. I think any cognitive, functioning individual would have recognized that this was unusual and a gift to be readily and eagerly accepted. And, since I was, I did.

The financial investment was serious money for a single female just beginning a metaphysical practice. Especially in a tradition with an Eastern philosophy which no one had ever known in the West. I was going out on a limb with only God standing below to catch me if I fell. Dr. Smythe was very kind and not only did I have two rooms, but his nurses would make my appointments and my clients could use his waiting room. After I became a Reiki Master he also let me use the center for my classes as well.

It was a boon for which I was very grateful.

As all the practical elements came together, I was clearly in my element. Dr. Smythe graciously taught me about professionalism in a health practice and the establishment of boundaries with difficult and demanding patients. To this day I owe him a debt of gratitude. I began telling people about this practice and they began telling others. I offered a free Reiki session every Thursday to those who had never experienced Reiki. As I was the first Reiki Master in the state of Texas, that was the majority of the population. Each Monday a Reiki clinic was offered. This provided the public with general information about this healing art.

Somehow during all this Suzanne heard about me and about Reiki. Suzanne was in her late twenties and a few years earlier had been involved in a car-train accident. Her two-year-old son, Bryan, was killed and she was left paralyzed from the neck down. Suzanne had experienced a difficult life prior to this accident, and her existence after the accident was worse. She had an abusive second marriage where her husband would yank her catheter out if she asked for water or juice. Luckily, Suzanne's parents were instrumental in ending that relationship.

An angel by the name of Janice walked into Suzanne's life. Janice was coming out of a difficult divorce, had training in nursing and needed a job. Suzanne, being totally wheelchair bound, needed someone to take care of her. This began Suzanne's experience with Reiki Touch Therapy. The drive from Suzanne's home to my office was well over an hour, but she came twice every week for double sessions of Reiki. Janice taught me how to place my feet onto Suzanne's feet, to lean backwards, pivot and turn Suzanne's body in order to lift and place her onto the treatment table. It was full body weight management and I gained great respect for physical therapists. Suzanne was sweet, beautiful and totally surrendered to the Reiki treatments. After all, it was years after the accident and no amount of surgeries, other therapies or medications had made any improvement in her quality of health, or her life, for that matter.

Even though Suzanne had no use of her hands I initiated her into the first level of Reiki so she would have the energy inside of her. I also initiated her attendant, Janice, so each time Janice touched Suzanne for any reason, Suzanne would receive the Reiki energy. In addition to the Reiki treatments we did guided imagery sessions, past-life sessions, etheric surgery and future-life sessions. In other words, we explored every possible avenue to provide a breakthrough for Suzanne.

One significant incident was the loss of Bryan. Suzanne could not forget or forgive herself for her son's death. She was haunted day and night by flash-backs and nightmares, torturing her body, mind and spirit.

Her anxiety and depression could not be managed with medicines. I suggested a future-life reading for Bryan. This would determine the status and the circumstances of his current existence. Suzanne was in such a guilt-ridden state she doubted that anything could be discovered but decided to proceed. I asked for Bryan's full name, his exact age at the time of his death and the location of where he was living at the time of the accident.

Using distance energy focusing with Reiki and combining it with an intuitive method called Integrative Awareness, I was able to reach Bryan's spirit. I saw him at about age eight in a room with blue painted walls in a two-story house with a window overlooking a very large lawn with playground equipment. He appeared very happy. I did not see any other children around and felt that he was an only child in this incarnation. There were photos of cars and also trains on his walls in the room. The cars were yellow, as was the car from which he was thrown. I had not previously known this. His name in this incarnation was Tommy, which I believe was his maternal grandfather's name. Tommy was subject to nightmares and was a loner. He was a handsome young boy and also smart but preferred being alone rather than having a lot of friends. I did not see his parents in this reading but understood that he was well loved and well taken care of. There were a couple of other pieces of information. He was wearing a blue shirt and had a blue blanket across the foot of his bed. This was in addition to his room being painted blue.

As I opened my eyes and looked at Suzanne, I observed two things. One was a look of joy and another were the tears flowing down her cheeks. Both were new for her. She had not experienced anything to feel joyous about, and her endocrine system had been dysfunctional since the accident, so tears were not possible. Even as Suzanne was clinging to the information she was also skeptical. She tearfully asked how I knew this was her little boy. This could be any little boy, anywhere in the world. She also wanted to know if he had experienced pain or trauma with the accident. It was a good and valid question. I asked her to let me take a moment to go back into the space of her son.

This time I went into the vibration of her son at the date of the accident. I asked him about the experience of being thrown through the windshield and his body impacting the train. Bryan's soul answered. The soul is very fragile. The soul knew it was about to leave this little boy's body. In order for the soul to stay intact for the next incarnation, it had to depart immediately before Bryan left the car. When the soul leaves, the body will feel no pain. The body is just a house or a space that the soul occupies while the body draws breath. So, Bryan felt no pain and his awaiting angels immediately took his soul.

Suzanne's other question was how did I know this was her son Bryan?

What if all this information was about someone else's little boy? She desperately wanted answers so she could be freed from years of pain and guilt. Her paralysis was payment for her being unaware of the oncoming train. I asked Bryan's soul for some piece of information, something that only Suzanne would know, so she could be assured of his new life and safety.

The soul asked for Suzanne to remember Bryan's little blue blanket.

I took another deep breath and opened my eyes. I related the information to Suzanne about the soul leaving his body. It greatly comforted and relieved her to know he had experienced no pain or trauma at the time of his death. She then took a deep breath and asked about her other question. How did I know this was Bryan and Bryan's soul, and that this Tommy in another life was her little boy Bryan? I reached over and put my hands on her hands. I looked into her waiting eyes and asked her if Bryan had a little blue blanket. Suzanne looked as startled as a paralyzed individual can. She lowered her head as more tears trickled down her face. When she was able to talk she said, "That was his 'blankie'; it was blue; he was never without it and he was buried with it; you found my son, and he is all right."

That was the beginning of a series of breakthroughs for Suzanne. Her angry, guilt-ridden body, mind and spirit melted into a happy, hopeful and future-oriented life.

New life was now happening all around Suzanne. Janice had not known a few months before, as she began work with Suzanne, that she was pregnant. Now there were babies in the house. Yes, babies. Two. Twins. Janice was certainly going to have her hands full. Suzanne's family was afraid Janice would leave because it would be too much work. Janice also did not know how she was going to manage two infants and Suzanne, too. The family pitched in and set up a schedule. The twins were probably a little confused as to just who the mommy was, because they were surrounded by caregivers. No one wanted

Janice or the children to go anywhere. Suzanne was delighted and the twins treated her like a mom, which made Suzanne very happy.

Now Suzanne elected to undergo etheric surgery. In her mind, there was every reason to have this experience and to engage in any activities that would improve her circumstances. Whether it is so or not, it appeared that her mental, physical and spiritual bodies were separated. It seemed that these bodies were not in synchronization. It certainly would be plausible that the impact sustained in the accident could have caused her energies to be out of alignment. There were many ways to approach this but Suzanne chose etheric surgery. She had earthly comfort wishes, such as driving a car, moving her arms and legs, complete healing of her spine, and also a relationship. She was a young, attractive female and did not want to be alone.

We invoked the presence of St. Germain, the Keeper of the Violet Flame. This Violet Flame transmutes, or changes, negative energy into positive energy. I did not then and do not now know of all the capabilities and attributes of the Violet Flame, but I have always had a fervent faith in this energy. It was imperative to gather and put into order, Suzanne's invisible bodies, to reinstate this cloak, if you will, of her energetic form. It was obvious that she was not together in this way. I felt that the conscious and intelligent heat of the Violet Flame would mold and frame a correct and functional order. It seemed best to work in this particular instance, from the outside in.

There were Violet Flames in the form of connecting cords that arose from Suzanne's physical body and began reaching out, in many and wide directions, to search for her invisible bodies. The first body, and closest to her physical form, is just that, her tangible, dense, physical self. Just above that is the etheric body. The etheric body contains everything the physical body has except for the density. Next is the aura body. Someone may ask you if you know the color of your aura, the color that is strongest from your chakra system. Just above that is the astral body, which is the abode for negative and positive energies, the home of free will in a manner of speaking, because our choices affect this astral body. The astral body will produce nightmares and fears as well as hopes and dreams. If someone is said to be astrally traveling, it is this body that can stay or leave. It is connected to the physical body by a silver cord and this cord is only severed at death. Next up is either the mental or the emotional body. This body can and does conform to the personality of the individual. If one is driven and governed by emotions and acts before thinking, then the emotional body is just above the astral body. If one is constantly analyzing and considering life before taking action, then the mental body is next. We are all ruled by one or the other, so these two bodies will be in a different layer with each individual. Next is the highest, the spiritual body.

You can see that we were asking St. Germain, with his Violet Flame, to perform a miracle. The flames were both discernable and hazy. I believe that is because I was not allowed to view all the methodologies employed in this endeavor. It did appear that the flames were sent out, rather in the manner of a fly fisherman, to hook the other bodies and to reel them in. Once they were in view, and I could see this, there were seamstress angels who very speedily sewed the bodies together. The thread was golden and glimmered with each stitch. The focus of the angels, as they performed this daunting task, was consummate.

Obviously I was merely observing this amazing feat. Suzanne was sound asleep on the treatment table. A new etheric leg was brought down, seemingly from thin air, and placed to the left side of Suzanne's left leg. This new leg, with everything needed except the new bone, was slowly introduced into the physical body space. The doctors used etheric tape, cut into five-inch long strips, about two inches wide. This tape was utilized to connect and tape together all the new components around the bone. After everything was in place, an etheric white mist completely surrounded the foot, ankle, knee and femur.

Next they moved to the spine. Using small silver knives with three-inch blades, the spine was rapidly but meticulously cleaned. At the fusion of the neck new pedicles were formed to provide movement. These new pedicles, or small projections from the vertebrae, were about one-half inch in size. Four spearlike instruments were positioned in place on four sides of this procedure. The spinal fluid was drained and new spinal fluid introduced. All processes included the white mist etheric wrap.

Moving around to Suzanne's left arm, the doctors skillfully opened it from the forefinger to the shoulder. The procedure was similar to the femur process, except the bones were not as shattered. Hours passed as if they were seconds. The doctors, in stiff, white coats and mirrored headbands, complete with lights, continued ceaselessly. The arm was rebuilt and the gluelike etheric, ectoplasmic substance held it in place, protecting and healing every cell. The etheric substance is Suzanne's. The ectoplasm is the life force necessary for bringing the healing processes to completion. Doctors Forrest, Murphy and Brown had delivered creative sculptured movements, the essence of perfection in each action.

They now looked at me. I knew this look. They were finished. And they were tired. Energy is energy and bodies are bodies, whether in form or not. As one, the three doctors took three steps back and disappeared into the ethers.

They would now rest, then go on to the next task somewhere else in the world. In my travels, teaching and performing healing work, I would encounter other healers who also had the great good fortune of working with these good and generous doctors.

I gently awakened Suzanne. I asked her how she felt. She had been still for about two or three hours. Half her body had been rebuilt. Neither of us knew why the left side was chosen and not the right side, but we accepted the wisdom of the doctors and were grateful beyond measure.

Suzanne was my client for about two years. She experienced all I knew to offer with Reiki Touch Therapy being the basis of each appointment. She also had the benefit of Reiki in her own body; and she had Janice and, later, the twins all eager to give her this energy too. A walking rail was built in the home for Suzanne. She had to face the wall and take very tiny steps. I encouraged her to return to physical therapy for guidance and strengthening. She could now feed herself, turn pages in a book and use a telephone. Her endocrine system kicked in and her menses, perspiration glands and tear ducts were all function- ing normally. Suzanne enrolled in college and was a brilliant student. Her fam- ily and friends marveled not only at the physical changes but also at the attitude and gratitude Suzanne now had for life. She was happy and had enjoyment with each day. She had forgiven herself. The guilt was gone and we had done further work for Bryan in his new body. With Suzanne's transformation Tommy also attained a new approach to life. He no longer had nightmares, became more gregarious and joined sports groups, just like a normal, active boy. He also added other colors and decorations to his room. His past seemed to fade away.

The transformation was of great magnitude all around. Some limitations existed. However, the overall change was nothing short of a new lease on life for Suzanne's body, mind and spirit, and for all those around her.

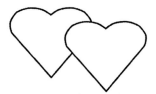

MEDITATION
Heart Cave Guided Imagery

There are multitudinous styles and forms of meditation. For those who do not practice it or know anyone who meditates, one looming question is: Why meditate? It takes time to meditate and why not just take a nap for the same benefit? Let's explore some avenues, approaches and reasons for meditation.

I have formally studied meditation for about thirty years. Many studies have documented the benefits of meditation. Meditation can aid in preventing the following: hypertension, coronary heart disease, stroke, ulcers, arthritis, colitis, diarrhea, asthma, backaches, muscle tension, temporomandibular joint syndrome and cancer. Stress is a major factor in most illnesses and meditation can and does relieve many symptomatic manifestations. As an adjunct professor of psychology I can attest that exam scores are higher and blood pressure is lower if the student meditates. These are a few maladies in which meditation can have a direct and positive effect. The benefit of having a more balanced and harmonious life is a plus, too.

Visual imagery is a form of meditation with a teacher guiding a student or client through this imagination process. In the next section, I will present some guided imagery sessions with clients. You may notice that, like other practices, this involves engaging the feelings of love and opening the heart to explore and heal various situations.

The heart is frequently a focal point with meditation. Some teachers discuss the heart both physically and metaphysically. Jean Houston, PhD, lectured about the physical heart having four chambers, then carried the class into a shamanic journey of the heart. Sometimes the back of the heart is addressed and known to be an area in which we may tuck our dark grudges or deep grief. The front of the heart is often depicted as having doors. Are your heart doors open or closed? One Great Being suggests that we go into this sacred space and roam. Ahhhhh.

The following is a Heart Cave Guided Imagery journey for a client. We will address her as Kathy. Kathy was having trouble with her marriage and was in a depressive state. After exploring other methodologies of healing, this meditative technique was approached.

Many times I perform Reiki Touch Therapy on the client for a half hour before the technique begins. Reiki brings balance and harmony to the body, mind and spirit, so the client is calmer and more receptive to the meditation. After Reiki the client moves to a chair for a comfortable seated position. I tell the client that it is better to have the eyes closed. I will have my eyes open and will be taking notes during the procedure. The client is allowed to bring a tape recorder if they choose. After a brief explanation of the entire process, we are ready to proceed.

Kathy's eyes are closed and I am ready to begin. I ask Kathy to take a couple of deep breaths, acknowledging her breath as prana, or divine breath. As she inhales and exhales I ask her to have gratitude for this process. Gratitude will enhance the process for smoothness and for more positive results. As Kathy inhales and exhales, I gauge my breath along with hers and deeply bring in the prana also. After this I instruct Kathy to begin her normal breathing pattern and just be comfortable for this journey into her heart. Notice the details in the instructions. Note that nothing is assumed or taken for granted.

I tell Kathy to picture herself in an ordinary room. I describe the room as having four walls, two windows and one door. I ask her to walk to the door, grasp the doorknob, turn it, open the door and walk through it. I ask her to securely close the door behind her. I ask her to tell me when she has done this. She verbally states that she has. I write all this down. I tell Kathy that in front of her are some stairs. There are ten stairs. There is a railing on either side for support. I tell her that I will count her down the stairs and that she is to begin with her right foot. Counting: one, two, three, going on down, four, five, six, seven, moving on down, eight, nine and ten. You are now at the bottom of the stairs. Directly in front of you is a door. This is the door to the cave of your heart. Carefully examine this door and when you are ready, describe it to me. Kathy says the door is nine or ten feet tall, is wooden, painted and in an old house. I ask her if she can see a handle with which to open this door, and to tell me what it looks like. The handle is a rusty brown doorknob. I ask her to open the door, walk inside and close the door securely behind her, then tell me when this is done.

Kathy is now inside her heart's cave and I ask her to describe what she sees. She says it is dark, but there is a light in the distance, that it has an aquarium-type atmosphere. There are dark corners with no light and she perceives a blackish red color. The left ceiling slopes upward and has a light high up on a rounded wall. There are no angled walls in her heart cave. I inform Kathy that this is her heart cave and that she can decorate it anyway she likes. So Kathy adds a skylight, some windows, a candle by the door to mark the exit and track lights for the dark corners. She adds a Renoir painting of children and a rocking chair. She adds some Dan Fogleman music then announces that it is all done.

I ask Kathy to create a comfortable seat large enough for her and one other person. Each time a request is made I ask her to inform me when it is done. She puts a thick and very soft lamb's-wool rug on the floor. I ask her to sit at the left and to leave the right side available for a Great Being of her choice. She chooses Christ to come and sit beside her for support. He enters, wearing a white robe and sandals, and greets Kathy with a glowing smile. She is also smiling, and I ask her to talk to me about this occurrence. Usually I can see everything the client sees, and the interchange of conversation keeps the energy flowing. As Christ gets comfortable on the rug, I tell Kathy to welcome Him and to tell Him why He is here. She silently explains to Christ that she is having marital problems and needs His support as she is guided through this process. He smiles in agreement and she returns the smile.

I ask Kathy to look in front of her. I tell her that she will see a stage, an ordinary Broadway-type stage. The stage has steps on the left and on the right. I ask her "unhappy body" to walk up the stairs on the left side and to stand on the left side of the stage. I ask her to tell me when she is there. She does. Kathy's "happy body" remains on the floor sitting beside Christ. I ask her happy body to take Christ's hand for strength.

Once Kathy's unhappy body is on the stage, and appearing most miserable, I ask her to talk about her problem. She talks to her husband as he is represented in her body. She says that she presents only pain and unhappiness to him and she knows that things are not like he had planned. That he has been unable to pursue his business endeavors because of her dependence on him. She discusses her despondence and depression and how she puts herself into the lives of their children. She says he constantly quizzes her about every moment of the day, and she feels he does not trust her. When he arrive home he goes to his office, closes the door, calls his mother and talks until dinner is ready. There is never any appreciation for dinner or any interest in the children's activities. She feels that she has not given him what he wants in a marriage and that she does not know what to do.

I ask Kathy to imagine and to create a very large container and to put it at her left side. She does this. It is a big cardboard box with a garbage compactor lining. I instruct Kathy to choose one of her problems and to put that problem into some type of tangible form. She chooses his mother and makes her into a green monster. I ask Kathy to put the green monster into the container. Kathy happily complied. I asked her to choose the next problem and to put that problem into a tangible form. The next was the psychological abuse, which she forms into a hammer. She puts that into the box. The other problems are conditional love, ignoring their children, deception regarding future dreams and plans, denial of emotions and many, many others. Each problem is attached to a tangible form and put into the box. At times I ask about the size of the container; if it is big enough or not. The size has to be enlarged more than once. Kathy has carried a heavy load for a long time.

I tell Kathy's unhappy body to remain in place on the stage. Now, I respectfully ask Christ to stand and to take Kathy's hand and for them both to go up the steps on the right side of the stage and stand there. I ask them to tell me when they are there. I relate to them that they will build a fire, a very large fire, as tall or taller than they. I show them the stones from which to form a circle so the fire will not spread. There are logs, kindling wood and matches to start the fire. Together they energetically, with great focus, build the fire. I ask them to let me know when it is as high as their heads.

I motion for Christ and Kathy to now retrieve the cardboard box and to drag it over to the roaring fire. I tell Kathy to reach in and pull out the first item, to tell me what it is, then throw it into the fire. The first one is her husband's mother, the green monster. Off she goes into the fire. I ask Kathy to let me know of any noises the objects might make. The green monster was not happy to be tossed into the fire. One by one, until the container is empty, all objects are named and tossed into the fire. Then, I tell them to lift the cardboard box, to turn it upside down and shake it, to ensure that it is, indeed empty. It is. Now they throw the box into the fire.

It is time for Christ and Kathy to move to the middle of the stage while the fire consumes all the unhappy body problems. I ask Christ to ask Kathy to state some positive desires she wishes from her husband. Kathy states that she wants the following: respect, eagerness and happiness for the relationship, emotional attachment, cooperation with raising the children, to make decisions together and for him to keep promises, to have a true marriage with caring and sharing, with a happy future together.

Now Kathy and Christ move to the left side of the stage where the unhappy body is standing. The unhappy body is an empty shell now, having gotten rid of all the unhappiness. Christ calls in some angels and He, the angels and Kathy join hands and move around in a circle, softly singing and praying for all Kathy's desires to fill the unhappy body shell.

Christ calls in the Sun and asks for the warmth and energy of the Sun; then He calls in the Moon and asks for the softness, the femininity and the glow of the Moon. When the unhappy body is filled, it is no longer the unhappy body. During the movement of Christ, the angels and the unhappy body, Kathy has merged with this empty shell. The empty shell is now inhabited with the happy Kathy.

Christ now takes the happy Kathy's hand and together they stride across the stage to discover that the fire has consumed all the objects in the container and the container itself. There are ashes left and a long stick is nearby. Christ points to the stick and indicates that Kathy should pick it up and stir the ashes. As Kathy stirs the ashes she feels something hit the stick. The ashes are cool so she reaches down and picks up the object. This object is a silver cross on a silver chain, to wear around her neck. This is a gift from the ashes for Kathy to wear all the time so she will be reminded of her work. She asks for Christ to assist her in putting it on. He does.

The complete and happy Kathy now comes down off the stage with her beloved Christ. She is a new person, endowed with many positive attributes. I tell her that it is time to thank Christ for His participation and to bid Him farewell. I tell her to watch until He is completely out of sight and to let me know when He is gone.

I now inform Kathy that it is time to leave her heart's cave and that she must go around and put out all the lights and candles. She may leave one on so it will be welcoming to her upon any return. After that is done I ask her to move to the door of her heart, to grasp the handle firmly, to open the door, move through it and to close it securely behind her. After that is accomplished, I reveal to her the ten steps that go upward and are directly in front of her. I tell her that I will count her up the stairs and for her to begin with her right foot.

You are going up the stairs now: ten, nine, eight, moving up, seven, six, five, four, going on up, three, two and one.

You are now at the top of the stairs. In front of you is a door. This is the door to the ordinary room. Grasp the doorknob firmly, open the door and walk through the door, closing it securely behind you. You are now back in the ordinary room. The room with four walls, a couple of windows and the door from which you just entered. Take two long, deep breaths, letting the exhalation out slowly each time. Then resume your normal breathing pattern and, when you are ready, you may open your eyes.

Kathy and I both could use a cup of hot tea now, so I prepare that as she gets back into her body. The first questions are, did that really happen, is that a real experience, and will it work?

The timing for it to "work" is different for everyone. I personally can attest to the fact that it does work and rather rapidly. The phenomenon of it is that it works on both or all parties. Something has shifted and action follows thought.

Reiki Touch™ Therapy Meditation

There are initiations in which an individual is introduced to the energy form of Reiki. In order for the student to optimize the reception of the initiation a meditation is done. These meditations take different forms as to length of time and variations of themes. The following is a guided meditation, which brings the student into a state of balance and harmony, as well as programming information into the body, mind and spirit.

Allow yourself to get into a comfortable position and gently close your eyes. Inhaling through your nose, take a deep breath, bringing the prana all the way down to your toes. Now, exhale slowly and long, letting the breath out through your mouth. Again, let us take a deep inhalation and add the element of gratitude to your breath. As the breath flows deeply within your body, mind and spirit, be grateful for this breath, this prana, this life-sustaining force. Whenever you are ready just resume your normal breathing pattern.

Reiki comes from the land of Tibet. Imagine that you are now in Tibet. See yourself standing on a very high mountain gazing down into a vast valley below. This valley stretches as far as the eye can see to the left and as far as the eye can see to the right. As you scan the valley you will see little villages dotted about, lakes with mists over them, many trees and animals grazing on the mountainsides. You are enjoying this beautiful sight with the serene and lush green scenery.

As you look to the right you observe that a mist has lifted off a lake. Just beyond the lake is a majestic, Tibetan Temple. Your heart leaps for joy, it is as if that view is what you are waiting for. You begin running down the side of the mountain, passing the grazing animals, maneuvering through the trees and villages, and finally, finally reaching the Temple. Slowly, with reverence, you go up the steps; one, two, three, four, five, six and seven.

As you reach the seventh step, you enter the Great Hall of the Temple. It is breathtakingly beautiful. The walls are designed with different colored woods carved into sacred symbols and embedded with precious gemstones. You walk over and, with great care, run your fingertips over the walls . . . and remember. Now, moving on down the halls, you pass a room with monks, sitting in rows, doing their daily chants. A little farther and you observe another monk tending to the gardens. The silence is tangible and you almost do not want to breathe.

Walking on you notice a room with a bright light coming out into the hall. You go over to this doorway and look inside. The room has books from the floor to the ceiling on every wall. In the center of the room is a long wooden table with chairs around it; and at the far end is a little monk. He is resting his chin in his hands, has a twinkle in his eye, and beckons for you to enter. With your right foot you enter this room. Immediately upon putting your foot inside you are aware that this is the Hall of Records for Reiki. Every word ever spoken or written about Reiki is here in this room. And one of these books is yours; your very own personal Reiki book. Find your book. Find your very own personal Reiki book. It will reveal itself to you. Perhaps it has your name on it. Maybe it is your favorite color. Your book may be nudged out away from the other books or it may just fall on the floor at your feet. In some way your Reiki book will reveal itself to you right away.

As you get your book clasp it to your heart, as if giving it a big, warm, welcoming hug. Fill your book with gratitude for coming back into your space. Take your book over to the long wooden table. Pull out a chair, take a seat and place the book on the table in front of you. Now, place your Reiki hands onto your very own personal Reiki book and again express your gratitude. Tell your book that you want it to reveal to you specifically what you need to know at this moment. You will have some time in silence to peruse your book. The little monk is there for you if you have a question. Take some time now, in silence, with your book. Open your book and begin. (Time: one minute).

You have now received, either subconsciously or consciously, whatever your very own personal Reiki book has to offer you on this auspicious occasion. Close your book now and, in your own way, offer your gratitude to your book as you replace it onto the shelf where you found it. The little monk is awaiting you now. Go over to the little monk and respectfully bow before him. Ask him for a message for your life. Wait a moment to receive it. If you do not understand the message ask the little monk for an explanation. Wait to receive it. Now ask the little monk for a gift that represents the message to you. Again, if there is a question regarding the gift you may ask its meaning. When this is complete, in your own way, offer your gratitude to the little monk for allowing you to come into the library, for the message and for the gift.

Go back to your chair at the wooden table. Pull it out and take a seat. Get comfortable to prepare for your Reiki initiation. With your eyes closed, contemplate your surroundings, the information from your book and the gifts from the little monk. Begin to breathe in your normal rhythm and prepare to receive the initiation.

After the initiation the students are invited to share any meditation experiences. The student is also assured that all information may be kept sacred within and sharing is not mandatory. The student is encouraged, if possible, to obtain the monk's gift in a tangible form to bring the energy of the message into a conscious state. For example, in my meditation the little monk gave me a red glass heart. To my knowledge, I had never seen one. In order to have something tangible, I drew it out in full color on some paper. One day, while shopping for something else, I happened to be drawn to a table that held some stationery paperweights. There it was; my little red glass heart! I was immediately transported back to the image of the little monk handing it to me. As he handed it to me he told me that hearts are as red as the fiery sun and also as delicate as glass.

There are many, many facets of meditating alone. This can involve breathing techniques, sitting or lying postures, certain room settings with light control, music or no music and other practices designed to enhance and augment meditation. Because of the various methodologies of meditation it is vitally important to have a teacher for proper instruction.

At the beginning of the chapter I offered the question, "Why not just take a nap?" There are many reasons to meditate instead of taking a nap. Some teachers say that one hour of meditation can equal the benefits of up to six hours of sleep. This of course depends on proper instruction of meditation techniques.

Many say that they do not know how to meditate. Meditation is an art as well as a spiritual practice and must be followed in form for the benefits to be effective.

Meditation Alone

Have a meditation mat—something upon which to sit. This should be a mat that no one else uses for anything. Lower the lights, have some soft, soothing music, light a candle and perhaps have some incense too. Use some small pillows to support your back and knees. Comfort is essential. Sit in an upright position with the spine straight but not rigid. Place your hands either in your lap or on your knees. Some individuals prefer a focal point so you may choose to gaze at the candle flame until you sense an altered or relaxed state within. You know that when you put your head on your pillow to go to sleep at night, that you do not instantly fall asleep. You have all these thoughts about the day, your family, your job and other occurrences. The same can happen with the first part of meditation.

Use the candle as a focus and allow the thoughts to just flow through your mind as you become calm and relaxed, and you'll soon drift into a sweet meditation. Even though you are surrendering to this state, it is different from sleep. Use your breath to carry you deeper into this state. Inhale through your nose and exhale through your mouth. Breathe very slowly and fill your body with the breath. Exhale as much breath as is comfortably possible. If you have a master meditation teacher or a Guru who has given you a sacred Mantra, then use the breath to bring the Mantra in and out with your breath flow. If you have a belief system that has some calming phrases, then use one of them. It might be as beautiful and as simple as "God is Love" repeated over and over with the inhalation and the exhalation.

Sally Kempton, in her *Awakened Heart* CD, brings the energy inside for a deeper and more relaxed state. As you begin to close your eyes, adjust your thoughts to your surroundings. Using the word "aware" very slowly become aware of your body from head to toe. Become aware of your head, your face, your neck, your shoulders, your upper and lower torso, your legs and your feet. When you have completed the awareness of the body, move on to an awareness of your body as it relates to your meditation mat, the music, the very air around you, the walls of the room, everything around you. You will have a deeper sense now of who you are in relation to the area. You will gain understanding of all that is, in this room and beyond, with an added understanding of being one with the universe. Now, this is worth meditating, wouldn't you say?

Time seems to lose itself, so have an alarm if you need to have a schedule for your meditation. If your posture is comfortable, the room is quiet, and your breathing is maintained you will have a calming experience. It is good to meditate in the same area of the same room, on the same meditation mat, with the same or similar music. The energy will build and you will discover that you will be able to fall into meditation easier and faster each time. It is good to begin and end a day with this practice. You will be more centered, more confident, more relaxed and have infinitely more peace of mind. There are many wonderful books about meditation. Read them, develop your own style and have a better life.

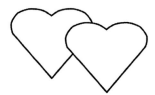

APPEARANCES & FORGIVENESS

I am choosing to use the word appearances in lieu of apparitions even though at times it may seem that the latter is the more apparent word. Appearances can occur if one is still in one's body on the earthly, physical plane, and we usually attribute the word apparition to one who has left their physical body and gone to other realms.

When my mother was about to leave her body, she began having dreams and visions of her dad, who had passed away some twenty years before. During this same time, while resting in the living room of my mother's home, I saw a photo of my paternal grandmother "come to life" and tell me that on the other side they were preparing for my mother's arrival. When I mentioned this to my dad, he discounted it, saying that he did not believe in communication from the dearly departed.

Oncology nurses have related these circumstances to me. One nurse was sure that her patient was going to survive his cancer ordeal until he began sharing some dreams he was having about his deceased aunt. These dreams were a sign to this nurse that he would be joining his beloved aunt.

After my paternal grandmother died, she appeared to me. It was late and she suddenly was standing at the foot of my bed. This is a common place for appearances to occur. She told me some things about my family. In return I asked her just what it was like over there and was she happy. She said that it was all right and she was happy enough. She had been blind for twenty years and said that now she was happy that she could see her relatives.

Before my maternal grandmother passed away, I had dreams of my mother, who left her body over ten years before my grandmother's demise.

My maternal grandmother came to me in several different forms after she died. First, her face appeared directly in front of mine. She held my face with both her sweet hands and smiled a golden smile, following that with kisses all over my face. She was the last of a long line of family to go and she was very happy to be there instead of here. Second, as I was coming out of a room, she stood, full body, stubbornly not moving, and shook her finger at me. She instructed me as to some property she had left for me but it was taken away and I would have to fight for it. I already knew that and had decided to let it go.

As is mentioned in a previous chapter, a young client, Dylan, bounced back and forth from my house to his immediately after he passed away. He had been with me daily for two years and therefore was very comfortable in my space. Everyone at his house was crying and calling everyone and making last rites arrangements. He said it was more peaceful with me. He sat at the end of my bed, even within a half hour of his passing. He sat cross-legged and asked a thousand questions. What was going to happen to his body? What clothes would they put on him for the funeral? Would his casket be opened or closed? Many, many questions. I told him he could wear whatever he wanted and the casket could be as he wished. I told him to tell his mother what he wanted. All during the night he came back and forth between my house and his house. He would be musing about his life and the next life, then suddenly say that he had to go check on his mom.

The more an individual is open to visits from other realms, the more often it will occur.

If there is concern, then do not feel you must do this.

Forgiveness

On an *Oprah* show a former Zen monk was discussing his hospice work and the last wishes of his patients. He stated that no matter how long the individual had been ill, in the last few days or hours of life there was one regret, one remorse. Out of almost a thousand patients all wished they had had the opportunity to ask for forgiveness for something, big or small, that they had done. They wanted to mend relationships, repair guilt situations from their former jobs, and to make peace with God.

Many individuals took this information and realized, especially after September 11, 2001, that extra effort was necessary to make this happen. I was one of them. The show was around Christmas time. So just after Christmas I sat down and made a list of everyone I knew. I had addresses, phone numbers and email accounts. I wrote a simple message to all. I said how much they had meant to me, in a specific way if that was the case. I related the *Oprah* show, the Zen monk's experience. I said that it moved me to ask for forgiveness and to make every effort to achieve a state of equanimity and peace with all those I knew. Hundreds were contacted. To my great pleasure most efforts were returned with lovely cards, gifts and exclamations of gratitude. Some were simple emails saying, "all clear here." But, not all. Some had real issues with me. I was unaware of it and would have gone to my death being unaware. I treated each issue with great respect. I either met with the individual in person or connected in some other way. I hope and pray that I reached them all and also realize that it would be a good practice to repeat each year, for the new people we meet every day.

Holding on to anger, hard feelings, vindictive natures and resentment can harm the body, mind and spirit in serious ways. It can alter a personality and affect everyone. The forgiveness can provide a lightness of being, a glow in the heart and clear a vision for dreams of the future. It takes courage, but we are a courageous creation. We have God on our side. We can do anything. Gratitude brings you everything. Consider forgiving, and don't forget yourself.

Bryn

Bryn called and asked me to come to the hospital because she was giving birth and had a concern about the size of the baby. I had participated in giving Reiki Touch Therapy in many delivery rooms and knew the obstetricians. The doctors had wavered between a cesarean section and a natural childbirth. There were many factors, one influenced by my client, who wanted a natural birth process. When her water broke it filled two containers. Because each container held a pound of water the obstetrician determined that the baby was actually two pounds lighter than expected so a natural childbirth was planned.

Twenty-three hours later both Bryn and the baby were in jeopardy. The vital signs were not registering normally and I knew everyone was very concerned. The baby had already been pushed, pulled and shoved into the birth canal so it was too late for the cesarean. No medications could be given because of the timing and the need to have some semblance of physical contractions. The doctor came out of the room and I followed. I asked her just how big was this baby. She said that a slight miscalculation revealed that the baby was over nine pounds and possibly ten pounds. There was nothing slight about the miscalculation. The doctor was of Hindu persuasion and I knew that her God was Shiva. I took the doctor by her shoulders and yelled, three times, "Shiva is delivering this baby, Shiva is delivering this baby, Shiva is delivering this baby."

I could tell that the doctor was in a state of shock and exhaustion as was her patient. I turned the doctor around and brought her back to Bryn who was in a very weak state herself. Time was of the essence. The baby had to be born immediately. Some emergency surgery was performed and the baby was born. Everyone immediately scurried around to make sure that proper medical procedures were available.

The baby was taken to the critical care nursery and Bryn was put into a room close by, across the hall from the nurses station. She had tubes everywhere: intravenous for dehydration, pain medications and antibiotics, catheters, and for the monitoring machines on all sides of her bed.

It seemed that she was all right for the rest of the night so I went home. We had all been there for about two days without sleep. I went right to sleep when I got home. Then a bright light wakened me. It came from the foot of my bed. I truly thought I was dreaming so I put my head back down on my pillow and closed my eyes. The bright light did not go away.

I sat up in bed and stared at it, really too tired to make sense of it. The light revealed a figure I recognized as Bryn. I asked if something was wrong. She said that she was leaving and that I should come to the hospital immediately.

In my exhausted and skeptical state I telephoned the nurses station. I said that I had a concern about my client and would they just peek in and check on her. They assured me that she was fine. I asked them when her vitals were last checked. The response was that if I was not a medical person they could not answer that question. I asked them again to please just take five steps across the hall, open the door and see how she was. They refused.

I got up and quickly pulled on my clothes, put an orange power object in my pocket, grabbed the car keys and literally raced to the hospital, ordinarily twenty minutes away. I got there in five. As I reached the nurses station about two in the morning, they laughed and said that I sure was a determined person. I walked into Bryn's room and looked toward her bed. I could only see the bottom half of her body and did not see that right away. For a moment I thought she must have gotten up to go to the restroom, forgetting that was impossible with all her tube connections.

Then, with a gasp, I realized that she was in the process of dying, of leaving her body. Racing around to the side of her bed, I put the orange power object into her hands. I thought I heard her say, "Thank you." I put my hands on her head to draw the vital life force back up into her upper body. After about two hours she moaned. I moved to her heart and solar plexus, or stomach area. After another hour her breathing seemed to stabilize. She put her hand over mine and very weakly, said, "Thank you, I knew you would come."

It took about four hours to bring Bryn back to a safe zone. At the end of that time she was smiling as the nurses brought her baby in for nursing. No one ever knew the trauma or the drama. She doesn't recall it either but thinks it is a nice story.

Angela

Then there was Angela. Angela was a twelve-year-old who overdosed on some of her mother's high-powered pain medications. Angela had been taking over a period of weeks, one or two pills out of the container. I had mentioned a depression notice to Angela and to her mother. Both discounted this information and completely declared that it was out of the question. Angela was bright and diligently preparing for cheerleader tryouts. No one seemed to notice that she was leaving her body. Her energy body was appearing to me, but since I saw her in person so frequently I too minimized this.

At nine in the morning her very anxious mother called me and asked me to do distant energy focusing for Angela. That morning her sister was unable to awaken her for school. Soon Angela's dad realized that her body was cold and yelled for everyone to get into the car and they raced her to the emergency room. Angela was pronounced DOA, dead on arrival. Her mother, an extraordinary woman, mandated that she was not dead and insisted on having her put into intensive care and hooked up to life support systems. The hospital called for psychiatric services, but they never came. To appease this distraught mother, they thought that they would just go through the motions and hook the child up to life support. The mother felt relieved and at that moment called me.

Naturally, I drove to the hospital. Angela was clearly dead. She was gray, cold, had no breath and the machines were registering a straight line. The mother said that she was in a coma and for me to begin doing Reiki Touch Therapy. I saw no reason not to accommodate her and felt that the energy might even help the child's transition from this world to the next. I did Reiki nonstop until late that night. It was a Friday. I set up a Reiki situational healing at home and that perpetuated all night. Angela's light body was very evident during the night, but she did not speak to me. By seven on Saturday morning I was back at the hospital. Angela's state had not changed; her mother had not left her side; the dad went to play tennis and to shop for a new sofa. Poor man, he did not know what to do. The look on the nurses faces indicated they wished they were also shopping or playing tennis.

I telephoned a child psychologist who dealt primarily with teen suicide issues. She arrived about one in the afternoon. The look on her face registered what everyone, except the mother, was thinking. That Angela was, and had been for some time, dead. We all had an unspoken contract with the mother to do what she wanted. And she wanted everything done for her daughter. Everything. Her stomach had been pumped. Charcoal had been introduced into her system. Other processes were ongoing.

The child psychologist drew up a chair and sat by the hospital bed. I was on the other side continuing the Reiki. The grandmother had arrived and was sitting with her daughter, trying to understand it all.

The child psychologist closely scrutinized Angela along with the rest of us in the room. In a moment I observed the psychologist register a look. I raised my eyebrows questioning her look. She whispered, "Angela's little finger just moved." We all know that the body can and does move after death so I did not take that as an important piece of information. The psychologist was determined to make me understand that the body had moved and that she thought Angela was alive. This was easily thirty-six hours after arriving at the hospital and the medications had been in her body for twelve hours before that. She had taken a dose that would have killed any adult.

Casually, I moved my Reiki hands to Angela's heart. Her mother noted this and cocked her head to the side as if asking if something was detected. I just smiled back with no concurrence. I felt something. I did. I felt a heartbeat. The psychologist motioned to the nurse to get the doctor. He came in and examined Angela; really just going through the motions. He saw no change and noted the support systems and machines had not altered. Somehow, we knew differently. After an hour or so the psychologist left but I stayed through the night. Angela's energy body appeared several times. She was smiling brightly but did not speak.

The next morning, Sunday, we were all going to have a face-to-face talk with the mother. We were kindly going to tell her that everything had been done, that Angela had made a choice, as tragic as it was, and the support systems should be removed. To our great surprise Angela opened her eyes and declared that she was starving. She went on to say, with all of us now standing and not believing what we were witnessing, that she wanted a cheeseburger, fries and a malt. Then, she said, two cheeseburgers! Her grandmother rapidly reached into her handbag, pulled out a candy bar and handed it to her. Angela ripped the wrapper off the candy and gobbled it up. The nurses ran in and tried to stop her from eating because of what the medications could have done to her digestive tract. And, besides that, she couldn't have revived. But she did.

Another nurse brought in a tray of liquid broth and some Jell-O, instructing Angela to slowly eat it. She explained to her that she had been in a deep sleep and had to take food very slowly. Angela consumed two trays of hospital food. That alone should have let us know that she was now fully awake and functioning. Her dad arrived, very happily, with bags of cheeseburgers, fries and malts. She consumed them all. Angela's mother happily collapsed from sheer exhaustion. Joy permeated the room.

Doctors from all over this huge medical center were brought in to check on this phenomenon. She would be fodder for research for her entire life. This was no ordinary miracle. Angela's vitals were so perfect that she was moved to a private room. I offered to stay the entire night so the family could get some much-needed rest. The next day was Monday and Angela wanted to go to school. No one agreed with her, so she watched television and talked to her friends on the phone all day. By that evening, the doctors, clearly perplexed, released her and also said they saw no reason for her to stay home from school the next day. Remember the cheerleader tryouts? They were on Tuesday. Did Angela try out? Yes. Did she win? Yes. To this day there are no known side effects. Angela is a beautiful and talented grown woman with a high value on life.

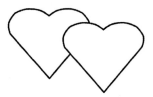

DOLPHINS

In the mid-eighties dolphins were very popular. People were flying to various sites to play and swim with the dolphins. A client of mine told me about a research site for dolphins in the Florida Keys. This was a center where I could not only swim with the dolphins but perhaps even experience some of the research. I was very excited.

I planned the trip and was to meet with an esteemed and practiced lady who was an expert with dolphins. Upon my arrival in Miami, my assistant, Kacki, apprehensively informed me that the dolphin expert had an emergency with one of the pods and had to leave for an undetermined amount of time. Disappointment was at a serious level. Kacki said that she knew I would not be happy at this turn of events so she got tickets for the Miami Aquarium Sea Show. My glance at her quickly registered my further dismay. She said for me to look on the bright side, there would be dolphins there; just not for me to swim with.

Reluctantly I agreed to go to this amusement park. What else was I to do? Go watch television in a hotel room? Go shopping? So, we went. There were several tanks where dolphins were swimming. We picked one and sat on the wet bleachers with the other tourists. After sitting there watching the trainer put the dolphins through their paces I noticed an empty bleacher to the side of the tank. I was guided to go there by myself.

As I watched the dolphins, I had the express impression that they were talking to me. I had planned on plying them with questions but they were ahead of me. This was true the entire journey. They were ahead of me. Me human, they water mammals! Or was that the case? One particular dolphin seemed to inquire as to the purpose of my visit. Intuitively a conversation ensued between us. I told him that I was a Reiki Master and wanted to communicate with the dolphins at the research center about how to work with dolphins and Reiki. The dolphin looked around because I was talking as if he were not a dolphin. I quickly apologized and expressed my disappointment that I could not be where I had planned. He assured me that he was, as well as the others there, a dolphin and could communicate with me just fine.

He asked me about Reiki and I told him. He nodded and said they were very familiar with Reiki and that it was known by them to be a great factor in bringing harmony to the world. My surprise at this remark was only superceded by all the other remarks and actions. I asked him if any of the dolphins, either there in Miami, or anywhere in the world, had been initiated into the Reiki energy. He sadly said that no Reiki Master had ever offered it. I was beyond thrilled and asked if I could have the honor. He said that there were fourteen dolphins in this tank and two other tanks on the premises with the same number and would that be too many? No indeed, it would not be too many.

With the distance energy focusing methodology, I asked that all dolphins in this tank who wanted to be initiated into Reiki Level I to please go to the ramp and be very still. They all went, put their heads onto the ramp and were silent and still as the process occurred. The trainer noticed that something different was happening. She had a bucket of fish and was wanting them to do tricks. Not now. After the completion of the Reiki I initiation the dolphins slid off the ramp and did a trick or two for the trainer, who was much relieved.

Now I asked if there were any dolphins in this tank that wanted to be initiated into the second level of Reiki. Seven dolphins swam to the ramp, placed their heads on it and became very still. They knew something stronger was being made available to them. I could sense their gratitude. I instructed them as to the use and the responsibility of Reiki II. Intuitively I could tell they already knew the great magnitude of this gift. Immediately after the initiation they slid off the ramp and happily splashed around. The energy had become so intense that a few tourists were looking over at me because they could feel some kind of connection.

For the final action I asked if there were any dolphins that desired to become a master in the lineage of Reiki. Only one did. He was the one with whom I first communicated at the tank. I instructed him in the duty and the vows of Reiki Mastery. Very slowly, as if in a procession going to a stage, he swam over to the ramp. The procedure was almost reversed. He told me what I was about to do before I did it. He knew the ancient secrets. He just had not had a Master to endow him with them. At the completion of this sacred ceremony he slid off the ramp. He seemed a little dizzy from the energy dispensation. I asked him if he was all right. He was very still. I observed him for a moment or two. Kacki came over and said it was time to go to another tank of dolphins and that we should go now. I put my hand up indicating one more moment.

I asked the Reiki Master dolphin to give me an unmistakable sign that he knew what he got and that he understood his new title and the responsibility of it. He was still then dove completely under the water. He soared up, all the way out of the water and gave a loud song of praise, like a shout to God. Then he came down full body and splashed the biggest splash of all. The audience thought he was putting on a show for them and they all stood and clapped. They were standing and applauding a new Reiki Master in a new realm. The new dolphin Reiki Master was humbled and pleased.

As we were leaving the tank the trainer came over and asked me what I was doing with the dolphins. She said she knew her dolphins and they were distinctly different this afternoon. I introduced myself and told her what I did, including the Reiki Master initiation for the one dolphin. She looked deeply into my eyes. She said, "The one with the Reiki Master initiation and the one with whom you communicated is Flipper, the famous television show dolphin." I was amazed and so pleased. My heart still warms at the memory of this experience.

Kacki and I went to the other tanks and other dolphins were initiated into the level one and two of Reiki. We left and had dinner, feeling we had contributed to raising the consciousness for the planet. I slept well, dreaming of dolphins playing in the moonlit ocean.

Early the next morning I was awakened by the ringing of the phone by my bed. It was a beautiful day. My assistant was calling to tell me that the dolphin research center in the Keys had contacted her to tell me to come on down there. The dolphin expert was feeling remiss that she had to be away and not meet with me, so she arranged for someone else to show me around. I was grateful and dressed quickly. Kacki met me in the lobby, and we delightedly sped away. The Keys are beautiful and serene. There was an aura of peace and calming in the air. I did not know if or how the joy in my heart could be any better than it had been yesterday.

We found the research center, went in and introduced ourselves. It was a very large establishment with many buildings, piers and separated areas for various research endeavors. Of course I wanted to swim with the dolphins, but it was not to be. This was not a swimming establishment, just research. The manager showed us around, going from one arena to the next, telling us all they were doing. It was too scientific for me and I will admit that I tuned her out.

As I walked from place to place I sensed three dolphins monitoring my movements. I asked the manager if I could rest a moment on this particular pier and she indicated that I could, just not to try to touch the dolphins. I sat very quietly sensing that some information was available if I could get into the right frame of mind. In my pocket, for some reason, I had three Herkimer diamond crystals. These are very tiny, double terminated crystals from upstate New York. I knew they had been cleared. I had no recollection as to why I put them into my pocket that day. Suddenly I was very aware that they were on my person and I pulled them out of my pocket. The dolphins were waiting for that very thing.

I put the three crystals in my palm and put out my hand so the three dolphins could see them. We all had a moment in time together. The dolphins were intently doing something to these crystals. I knew not what.

During part of this time the dolphins would switch positions in the water and before it was all over each one had been in the center between the other two.

I asked the manager if I could have a few more moments to rest and said that I might close my eyes if that was all right with her. My assistant knew I was about to do a cell memory process with the dolphins and quickly engaged the trainer in conversation. I did do the cell memory process and in that process asked the dolphins what they had just accomplished with me or with the crystals or what. They informed me that they had imprinted into each crystal, a matrix of the planet as it would be in one hundred years. I have seen and experienced so much in my life that I sometimes wonder why I am constantly amazed at Reiki and at life. This was definitely a time to remember, and I was then and am still amazed at this venture. I asked the dolphins just what I was to do with these crystals and the information now embedded in them. They told me to keep them; that at some time I would know what to do with them. I still have them and I still do not know what to do with them. Do you?

For relaxation Kacki had planned a side trip to the Everglades. This is a huge swamp. The beauty of all swamps is the misty, quiet, mysterious nature of the unknown. A different world really. There was a restaurant along the way, which served everyone on a big porch overlooking the wetlands. The view was very different and one almost had to adjust one's mental judgment as to the definition of beauty. Some very long-legged cranes strolled by in the tall grass. We did not pay that much attention to them and just continued to eat our lunch. We noticed that the cranes were not feeding in the shallow water but were intently watching us. Kacki wondered if they, like the dolphins, might benefit from Reiki. My mind first measured the importance of a dolphin next to a crane and in my mind the cranes fell way low on the scale. Error of understanding.

The cranes were beautiful and stately in their own way and it was clear that they wanted something. So I set up an intuitive communication conduit and asked what they wanted. They said they had been waiting a very long time for me and for the Reiki I could give to them. I was duly chastised and very humbled. Of course, I would initiate these cranes. And I did not only those but all we saw. A few stood out very clearly as teachers, and became crane Reiki Masters. It felt right. How I was going to explain it to my friends was another matter entirely!

Kacki and I drove on, ecstatic about the new drama unfolding with Reiki and its creatures. During the day, we encountered pelicans, other wild birds, snakes and even alligators. We let them decide. If they followed us around and pulled on our energy, they were initiated into Reiki. At a souvenir shop we purchased a map of the Everglades and initiated the entire area. While driving back, there was this enormous connection of being one with the universe. We had a cognizance that all were created and all had a purpose on the planet. Since that time, close to twenty years ago, whenever a crane, a pelican or an alligator is near me I have the distinct sense that we are connected with the Reiki energy. I do feel certain that the Reiki Master dolphins, cranes, pelicans and alligators are doing their duty and initiating other like beings into Reiki. I certainly now have a greater reverence for all creatures great and small.

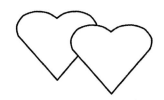

CHAKRA BALANCING

A ncient scribes and artists depicted energy systems of the body and named them chakras. These are described in modern texts but are derived from ancient belief systems. Even though there are major and minor chakra numbers and locations there are basically seven chakras or energy systems in the body. The major ones begin at the base of the spine, the root chakra, and go to the top of the head, the crown chakra. These are the ones addressed in this chapter and in the overall book.

As a Reiki Master, I use Reiki as the base of all healing modalities and methodologies. Beginning a chakra alignment or balancing, I first do hands-on Reiki treatment for ten to fifteen minutes on each chakra area.

Reiki balances and harmonizes the body, mind and spirit so this is a good beginning for any holistic system.

Each chakra or energy center has a color, an attribute and is located in a specific area of the body. When the color is particularly strong it will emanate away from the body, sometimes significantly. When this is discernable outside the body this is an indication of your primary or strongest aura.

Our chakras must be integrated for our system to be healthy and functioning. There are many ways to achieve this. Certain initiations from certain masters can provide it, meditation can do it and when necessary, a healer trained in the process can also achieve this integration. Traumas can put the chakras out of balance. Karma from this or another life experience can also cause an imbalance.

When a client comes to my office for a chakra alignment, there are several requirements for the optimum treatment. I will describe how to set up for this and will also give one or two instances of what may occur with the client.

The room is always "set" for healing. The lights are soft, the music is low and steady, water or tea and tissues are available and the treatment table is comfortable. There are plenty of cushions, pillows and blankets to ensure the security and comfort of the client. I use bright white sheets for chakra alignment. The colors are easier to detect this way.

The client fully reclines on his or her back. After the Reiki processes are completed, I stand at the client's solar plexus or stomach area. I put my hands at my third eye in a prayer-type position and ask for grace and guidance from a Higher Power. A protection method is also done to protect against any energies that may be released from the client during the process.

My hands are widely spread out to encompass the client's head and feet. I focus better with my eyes closed. I inform the client that their eyes can be open or closed but to please refrain from conversation during this procedure.

I begin to communicate with the various bodies because I have to enter and penetrate these invisible bodies to reach the chakras. I receive permission to enter the space.

With my hands spread wide, mentally enveloping the physical body, I ask the physical body for a word, a picture or a feeling that sums up or assesses the physical body state. The answer comes immediately.

Then I bring my hands inward, about six inches. I ask the etheric body for a word, picture or feeling which will give me the status of the etheric body. The etheric body contains all the components and information of the physical body but it is a faster energy because it does not have the density of the physical body. Again, the answer comes immediately.

Now, I address the aura body for a word, picture or feeling that sums up the state of the aura body as a whole. I am not, at this time, addressing each chakra individually. As I receive the answer I bring in my hands another six inches and address the astral, the duality body, and ask the same question so I'll have an idea of the condition of the astral body. The astral body is where negatives and positives can collide, resulting in tempers, nightmares or night terrors, and personality changes.

Bringing my hands in another six inches or so, I address either the mental or the emotional body of my client. If I perceive that my client is guided more by emotions, then I address the emotional body next. If my client is very mental and analytical, I will address the mental body next. This seems to change with each client. I request a word, picture or feeling and note that act so I will know the state of that body. Then I address the body that is next, either the mental or emotional.

The last body is the spiritual body. My hands are back together at the solar plexus area, but placed at my third eye again in a prayerlike position. I ask for a word, picture or feeling which assesses my client's spiritual state. After the information is received, I bow to the client's bodies and offer gratitude for the information.

At this time you may discreetly share with your client the information received. This is the healer's choice to do this now or at all.

If I choose to share, I usually do it with my eyes closed because I can remember the information more accurately. However, if I have a novice client I may want to observe the reaction to the information and will open my eyes. The reason you might be discreet is that the information is almost always symbolic and is the client's information. You, as the healer, do not know what the symbols represent, but the client usually does or a realization comes to them later. You have the ability to go into each symbol, but you have to decide if it is appropriate at this time to do so. Will this information prevent your client from staying open during the chakra alignment process? A separate reading can be arranged for an explanation of these symbols, but for now you have enough information to proceed with the chakra alignment.

You are ready now to proceed with the next step: going into each chakra one at a time. It is a good time to check on your client's comfort, have a short break, walk around a few minutes, have a drink of water or tea. It is good for the healer, too. A long process is about to begin. You thought it was over? Not yet.

When the client is positioned in the same posture as before, you are ready to continue. Go back to your original position at the solar plexus, again placing your hands at the third eye in a prayerlike position. Again, ask for guidance and protection, remembering that you are the vehicle, the facilitator for the information. The information is not yours; you are not making it up or imagining it. You are stating what you hear, see or feel from the client's energy sources. This takes away from your own ego situations and also prevents burnout. If you had to store all this information you would not last very long. Trust me on this.

Spread your hands out again toward the head and feet respectively, mentally encompassing the entire energy of the body, mind and spirit. Beginning at the head, ask the crown chakra for a word, picture or feeling that describes the state of that chakra. The answer comes immediately, sometimes almost before you ask, but do ask. Bring your hands in about six inches just as you did with the assessment of the invisible bodies and inquire as to the state of the third eye, the same way you did at the crown, asking for a word, picture or feeling. Each of these areas takes a maximum of five minutes. Move on down to the throat, the heart, solar plexus, sacral plexus and the root chakra area. You are bringing in your hands about six inches each time, following the same question procedure. When you are finished with all the stated chakra areas, your hands should be back over the solar plexus area. Now place them again in a prayerlike position and offer gratitude for the information.

The chakras work together, as does our body, mind and spirit. The first and sixth chakras correspond, the second and fifth chakras correspond, and the third and fourth correspond. For aligning and balancing, begin with the first three: root, sacral plexus and solar plexus. These are known as the lower chakras. Stand at the sacral plexus, the abdominal area, and put your hands in a prayerlike position at your third-eye level. Ask for grace, guidance and protection for you and your client.

Now, with your hands at your third-eye level, put your forefinger tips and thumb tips together, forming a triangle. Keep all fingers straight and firm. All. As the hands form a triangle, think pyramid, three-dimensional. Ask for Divine energy to blend with your skills. Experience this energy coming from the Higher Source universe, through your own crown chakra, through your third eye, going from your third eye into the triangle/pyramid within your hands. You may perceive or visualize this as an energy vortex, swirling clockwise as it enters your crown chakra and follows through into your hands. This is a powerful, whirling, "make it happen" energy.

With this vibrating, pulsating energy churning around in your hands, slowly and with great honor to the client's temple, lower your hands, still in position, about a foot above the three lower chakras. From your shoulders down, move your entire arms in a clockwise motion. Stay within the boundaries of the three lower chakras. Allow the pyramid in your hands to tumble or roll, extremely slowly, in a direction away from you, into the area of the three lower chakras. The pyramid is gently, but powerfully, plowing into the chakra space, sweetly encouraging the chakra to move into its correct direction and position. Make the clockwise circles wide, about a foot on either side of the body sides.

Move downward a bit, to just above the body, so the pyramid is tumbling one half outside and one half inside the body. You have just entered a heavy, dense energy so the focus is important. Notice the sluggishness of the movement. Breathe with the motion, focusing on your hands moving in a clockwise manner and the pyramid tumbling between your hands. Every now and then glance at your client's face. Their eyes are usually closed. Generally this is a procedure that does not bother them, but some are sensitive and may know exactly where you are and feel the motion in the body. Upon completion of the circle of one half in and one half out, submerge the entire pyramid into the body, guiding it above the body with your hands. Use the breath to gently go deeper with each circle. Spiral in toward the center of the abdomen before going to deeper levels.

Now, you may be wondering just how many circles must be made in each level? The answer basically depends on your focus and the crystallization or stuckness of the client's energy. I would say a minimum of three times, once for the body, once for the mind and once for the spirit. However, do not leave until the energy is flowing easily and smoothly in a clockwise direction.

Lower your hands to where the pyramid is one half inside the body and one half outside the back of the body; then completely outside the back of the body about a foot away. With each level, hands move clockwise and spiral from the outside to the center, or from circumference to the center.

The next step is to hold your hands above the sacral plexus area and have your left hand go to the crown in a circular, sweeping motion and return to touch the right hand. As the right hand is being touched it goes to the feet and returns to touch the left hand. Do this motion a total of three times, while silently repeating "as above, so below" each time. You are actually making a figure-eight motion. Bow to the three lower chakras and offer gratitude for the work.

The following chakras are done separately and individually. Put your hands, in the pyramid position, back at your third-eye level. Maintaining the position, move to the heart chakra region. Put your hands just over this area. Again ask for grace, guidance and protection for you and the client. Follow the same exact procedure as just done with the three lower chakras. Remember to place your hands, in the pyramid position, at your third eye before addressing the remainder of the chakras. And, of course, offer gratitude to each chakra when completed. From the heart you will move to the throat, then the third eye, then the crown. For these last three, the throat, third eye and crown, close your fingers and hands together to form a much smaller triangle and pyramid. The third eye, for example, would be almost thimble size. Just press your thumbs up into the finger area and you will have a smaller triangle.

The third eye is an area of which you may not be aware. Draw an invisible line straight in from between your eyebrows to the center of the head. Draw another line from your temples (side of your head in front of your ears) straight into the center of the head, draw a third line from the top of the head down to connect with the other lines. This is your pineal gland; your third eye. The outer physical opening is between your eyebrows.

Follow the procedure, going all the way from each chakra down to the feet with the triple repetition of "as above, so below."

For the crown, you move from the side of the client and now stand at the top of the head with the body stretched out in front of you. Follow the procedure of all the others and with the breath guiding your hands, send the energy all the way to the feet, again silently repeating "as above, so below."

For the close of this procedure, place your hands in a prayerlike position and walk from the crown to the feet of the client. Do not touch the client now. Have your hands a few inches away from the body. Walk back to the crown of the client and repeat this for a total of three times. Facing the client, step backwards until you are about six feet away. This moves you out of the healing energy space. You sit and observe your work. Observe each chakra, communicate with it, notice the depth and brightness of color and the direction of the flow of energy. This can take about twenty minutes, perhaps less. You may take notes if you desire.

Very gently bring your client back to an awareness of the healing atmosphere. They are in a fragile but strengthened state. After a brief and quiet conversation they may leave. I prefer to have a driver take them home; if they do not have a driver available, I do the process in their home. And I prefer to do this procedure in the evening so retiring for the day is a natural occurrence. The best case, energetically, is for them to sleep alone that night. Insist that the client rest and not get on the telephone, computer, or go to work, to a restaurant or shopping after this process. Otherwise, just do not do the process and realize this client is not serious about their wellness. Have two or three follow-up general healing sessions to ensure the stability of the work. If one has been trained in distance energy focusing, this can be done absently, without the client being physically present.

Following are some tiny excerpts and experiences with chakra alignment.

FIRST - Bodies:
> Physical — image of fetal position in a paralyzed state.
> Etheric — foglike envelope keeping everything intact.
> Aura — scrambled and mixed energy; lots of crossed lines.
> Astral — laughter at the energetic control of the client.
> Mental — black and white; divided vertically from head to toe.
> Emotional — budding, opening flower.
> Spiritual — sun behind a mountain; climbing the mountain to fully see the sun.

SECOND - Chakras:
> Crown — wooden jigsaw puzzle; splintered and jumbled.
> Third Eye — three-dimensionally open; would not or could not close, causing disturbance of discrimination.
> Throat — gurgling, bubbling, dark, oil-like substance
> Heart — Four chambers imploding; front was cracked emerald stone; back of heart was black.
> Root, Sacral Plexus and Solar Plexus respectively—imploding, closed, protective; indecision; script saying "do this, do that."

THIRD - After the chakra alignment: all moving in clockwise direction.
> Crown — gold and swirling in clockwise motion.
> Third eye — able to open and close at will.
> Throat — nectar.
> Heart — pure emerald in all four chambers, front and back of heart.
> Solar Plexus, Sacral Plexus and Root respectively—bright yellow sunrays; orange creation power restored; red balanced and in control.
> All bodies integrated and functioning in proper energetic order.

The aura is an outer manifestation of the color of each chakra. With some individuals these aura colors can be seen by a person experienced in this art. For instance, the color blue is around the throat and many teachers will have an exaggerated color of blue in that area. You can study the chart of the chakras, the colors and the attributes in this chapter.

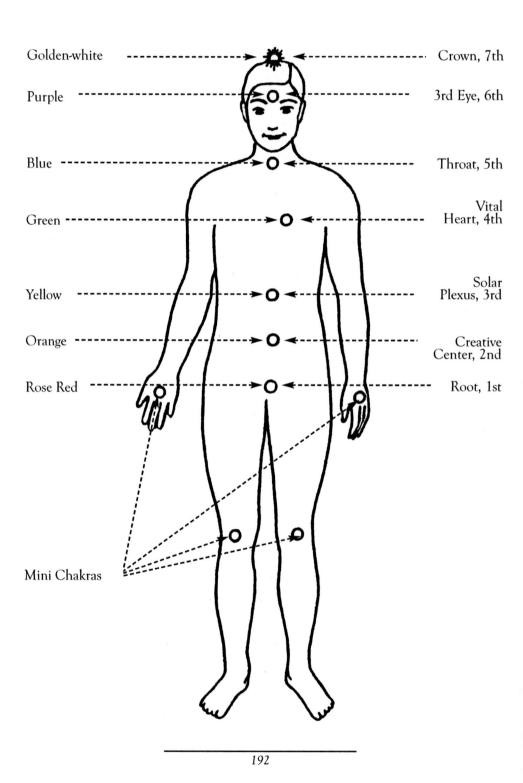

Golden-white · · · · · · · · · · · · · · · →   ← · · · · · · · · Crown, 7th

Purple ·   3rd Eye, 6th

Blue · → ← · · · · · · · Throat, 5th

Green · · · · · · · · · · · · · · · · · · · → ← · · · · · · · · ·   Vital
Heart, 4th

Yellow · · · · · · · · · · · · · · · · · → ← · · · · · · · · · ·   Solar
Plexus, 3rd

Orange · · · · · · · · · · · · · · · · · → ← · · · · · · · · · ·   Creative
Center, 2nd

Rose Red · · · · · · · · · · · · · · · → ← · · · · · · · · · ·   Root, 1st

Mini Chakras

COLOR CORRESPONDENCES

SOUND	COLOR	MUSICAL NOTE	PLANETARY INFLUENCE	HARMONIUS QUALITIES
E	Red	C	Mars	Determination, will, strength, activity, alertness, initiative, independence, inspiration and leadership.
O	Blue	G	Venus	Love, wisdom, gentleness, kindness, compassion, forgiveness, trust, cooperation, sensitivity, patience.
ă	Yellow	F	Mercury	Mental discrimation, evaluation, ability, joy, expression, joy, ability, expression, discipline, praise, sincerity and harmony.
A	Green	F	Saturn	All of the qualities of yellow and blue exist in green plus enthusiasm, responsiveness, acceptance, sharing, growth and expansion.
ĕ	Orange	D	Sun	All of the qualities of red and yellow exist in orange plus illumination, courage, analysis, victory, confidence, intellect, inventiveness, assertiveness and self-motivation.
U	Violet	B	Jupiter	All of the qualities of red and blue plus mercy, devotion, responsibility, loyalty, justice, idealism, wisdom and grace.
OM	Indigo	A	Uranus	Synthesis, inspirational, ritual, implementation, catalyst, aspiration, unity, balance, world service and humanitarian.

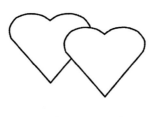

SHAMANISM

There are many doorways through which the life journeyer will travel. The Shaman enters into the inner realm. This entry, and its exit and the journey within, is intended to clear the pathways and to create or restore harmony and balance in an individual's life process.

A Shaman may employ drama, humor, struggle and other dynamics in the quest of successful restoration. Shamanistic healing covers a gigantic area; virtually all healing outside of the traditional or Western medical profession could be described as shamanistic. The appreciation and acceptance of this art depends on both the Shaman and the participating individual. The value of the practice rests solely on the shoulders of the patient and the Shaman.

There are vast stores of information regarding Shamanistic healings based on practice, psychology and science. The following journeys depict a dragon. The dragon becomes what you make it. The success of what the dragon does is dependent on your integration and acceptance of the journey. I invite you, as you read the following pages, to follow the instructions, to participate and judge the results for yourself.

DRAGON WORKSHOP
(SUPPLIES: crayons, paper, soft music)

I n our Western culture, a dragon is something to be slain, perhaps by a knight in shining armor. However, in the eastern cultures, the dragon is considered a benevolent being with good intentions, pearls of wisdom and endowed with divine powers.

We are going to explore the idea of an Eastern dragon, a good dragon that can slay our enemies, such as depression, anxiety, stress, anger and whatever else is negatively affecting you.

> We can all think of an image of a dragon.
> Is this a scary image for you?
> How does it make you feel?
> Close your eyes for a moment, take a couple of deep breaths.
> Now, think of a dragon, a powerful dragon, with good intentions to help
>   you slay your inner enemies.
> What does your dragon look like?
> What size is your dragon?
> What color is your dragon?
> If you could design your very own dragon to destroy your inner enemies,
>   what would it look like?
> Take a moment and mentally design your own special dragon.
> Take another deep breath now and come back into the room.

We are going to have an opportunity to create on paper our own personal dragon. You may design your dragon any size and any color, keeping in mind this is a good dragon and will do wonderful things for you.

As you create your dragon, firmly believe that this dragon has your best interests at heart, and will do anything to make you a healthy, more balanced person. While you are drawing, think of a name for your dragon. You may even ask your dragon what name he or she would want.

Note: Make sure everyone has paper and crayons; a tissue box could be handy. Walk around the room and interact as necessary.

Later: Now that everyone has finished drawing his or her own special dragon, just take a moment to look at it and begin communicating with your dragon. What kind of sound does your dragon make?

Start making sounds like your dragon. Get up and walk or crawl around the room, sounding and moving like your dragon.

Let us sit back down with our dragon.

Get into a comfortable position.

Close your eyes and take a couple of deep breaths.

Going deeply inside now, what inner enemy would you like your dragon to slay for you?

What is it that keeps you from optimal functioning?

Consider your dragon as your best friend whose only duty is to take care of you. That is the reason for his/her existence.

• Eyes still closed

Your dragon wants his or her own special position on your body, a place where he or she can have a clear view of you and your needs.

So, place your dragon on your right shoulder. Miniaturize your dragon so it will fit on your shoulder. Now, think of your inner obstacles, such as grief, anger, fear, anxiety, depression or whatever burdens you have now. Know exactly where in your body these obstacles, these imbalances, are. When you know exactly where they are, give them a form, something tangible. Be very clear what your obstacles look like.

• Eyes still closed

Now, calling your dragon by its name, gently invite it to come inside your body and carefully guide it to the first obstacle. Be very grateful while your dragon is destroying your enemies. Remember that your dragon is your very best friend and has only your highest interests at heart. Your dragon has sacred powers and can and will do whatever it takes to make you balanced in your body, mind and soul. When your dragon has devoured your obstacle a void is created, so put something beautiful into that void. It may be your favorite color, a flower or something special known only to you. You may want to place your hand over the area to seal or reinforce it.

Guide your dragon to the next place, always expressing gratitude, as your powerful dragon consumes the next enemy. When there is a void, just fill it with something pretty and, if you choose, seal the area with your hand.

Continue through your body, your mind and your soul until your very own personal dragon has removed everything that has kept you from functioning at an optimum level.

Take a couple of deep breaths and whenever you are ready just open your eyes.

We are going to divide into groups for sharing.
• <u>After the sharing:</u>
Remember that your dragon is always, with you, to help you at anytime.

Your dragon is for you alone. To be honorable, do not ask your dragon to work on other people.

Call your dragon by name, talk to your dragon, ask questions, go through this process as many times as you need to ensure the balance of your body, mind and soul. And always remember to be grateful.

DRAGON WORKSHOP Copyright Julia Carroll, 1987

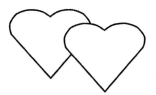

NATIVE AMERICAN LORE
Julia

Any caring and conscious individual now speaks of the Native American with great respect, and yes, even awe. Our heritage from the Native Americans is just that, our heritage. Yet, what have we done with this heritage? There are no caring or conscious words that would describe what we have done. Honor is not one of the words. Neither is respect. We have had a select few movie stars, political figures and some historians to endeavor to raise our guilt level to a degree of dignity. These have been short lived. The token "gift" of casinos on the reservations of the Indians are actually an insult. A culture and creed cannot be beaten down for centuries and be given crumbs in an attempt to establish equanimity. The Native Americans could have provided a roadmap for we "New Americans," but we took their land and imprisoned them in reservations. An attack such as this by the New Americans would have made any other culture extinct. Not this one. An attack by the New Americans would have caused any other culture's gifts to be erased. Not this one.

The Native Americans have a spirit that cannot be killed, no matter how vengeful the attack, how brutal the imprisonment or how much they continue to be abused and terrorized. We can and should, count ourselves fortunate that the Native Americans still have their culture, their ceremonies, and their rituals. The foundation of life itself is found within the spirit and knowledge of the Native Americans.

I was fortunate in my search for self, to have many encounters with our sacred Native American culture. The experiences cover the gamut, from common sense to the supernatural. I think, to the Native Americans, it is all the same. My daughter was studying Native American "Indians" in grammar school and upon exploring the territory within a hundred miles of her school, we discovered an Indian Reservation. One Saturday we drove to this reservation. There were no bright lights, no big signs saying, "Here You Are," no one "in costume" to entertain us. We even wondered if we were in the right place. We found a clearing on the land where it seemed that it was okay for us to park the car.

Nothing was paved, there were no sidewalks, certainly no McDonald's, and basically nothing going on. We came upon some one-story, unpainted buildings. There were a couple of men sitting on a bench and we wondered if they were "real" Indians. The clothes on their backs were tattered and out of fashion and the shoe styles were also from a few decades back. We were a bit uncomfortable. I asked one of the men if there was a souvenir shop or a place to get a cold drink. He stood, quite tall actually, and grinned widely, revealing many missing teeth.

He spoke the English language very well. I do not know exactly what we were expecting, but clearly not this. He took us inside and opened an ancient Coke machine and pulled out two bottles. They were room temperature and I noticed there was no electrical attachment to it. Actually were no electrical anythings around. It was as if we had stepped into a time very long ago; another world. He opened the bottles of soda and cheerfully handed them to us. I offered him some money and he took it. I recall being very glad that he took the money because abject poverty was evident on all sides.

We told him that my daughter was studying his people and that we heard there was a reservation there. We asked him if there was anything else we could see so she could write her school report. He smiled. This smile was so deep. It was obvious that we could not "see" what was there. We could only see what was not there. He informed us that in another month or two a play was being staged. This play would depict the history of the tribe. He also said, very proudly, that on that day some special dances would be performed in the native costumes. Other than that, no activities were planned. The area was in the middle of thick, dense forest. We were a young woman and her female child, yet we felt no fear. These were gentle, good-hearted folks. We thanked him for the sodas and drove away. My daughter and I were silent during the trip back home. There was much to contemplate. More than we knew.

Years later a group was going over to another town where these same Native Americans were holding a "sweat." A sweat is an event where a "sweat lodge" is built from scratch, fires are built, medicine wheels are put into place and ancient lore is revealed. The honor of the land seems to be the basis of the Native American experience.

There were about ten of us in the group. We had our Sony headsets playing rock music, had food and drink in the coolers and some other items such as a bathing suit and a blanket and towel. We had not a clue. We were unclear on the concept.

One Native American, a real one, was there. I say "real one" because we had no idea what to expect. His color was reddish, but otherwise he looked fairly "normal" to us. He was doing this for a couple that owned the land and they were doing it to bring blessings onto the land and for personal reasons.

The Native American and the couple were very busy. The intent was for us all to get very busy, too. Pronto. There was work to be done and I can tell you that no one knows authentic work more than a Native American. There were some shovels, some saws, wheelbarrows, old rags and other items to indicate work. We did not know this part, but we had traveled a few hours to get there, so why not pitch in. I am telling you this, dear reader, to educate you in the ordinary lack of knowledge of our heritage. Our attitude was not part of the heritage. We had much to learn.

The sweat lodge had to be built. There were stones being put into a pit, and other stones were being placed in a circle in another area of the land. To build the sweat lodge we had to tromp through the woods and find tall, lean saplings and cut them down. A precise number of saplings. I soon learned that the precise number of everything had much to do with Native American lore, or history. As we pushed our way through the woods, the guide, our personal Indian, taught us many things. We had to ask each sapling if we could cut it down. We had to tell the tree just what it would be used for. If a spider web crossed the path, we must take another path. We thought that he did not want the spider killed, but it was not that at all. If a spider's web crosses a path it is a warning that danger lurks ahead. We definitely took another direction. There were pine trees that would provide emotional strength and oak trees for mental courage.

We finally had the correct number and the right length of saplings, not to mention bug bites and scratches from the brush. The saplings were dragged out of the woods. Now they had to be tied together to form a dome and secured to the ground. Okay. After that there were old, very old, pieces of carpet, blankets and plastic tarp that were placed over this frame. The idea was to let no light come into the sweat lodge and to keep all the heat from the rocks in.

Oh, yes, the rocks. The pit was round and had a certain depth. Chants to both honor and encourage the fire lifted up into the heavens. There were a precise number of rocks and each rock had a name. There was a sequence as to when and where each rock was placed in the fire.

There was a chant for the rocks too. There were fire keepers and rock keepers. The fire had to be fed with wood (after permission was obtained from the wood), and the rocks had to be red hot and glowing to go into the sweat lodge. Permission was asked of each and every item used in the sweat process.

Another pit was being dug in the sweat lodge and the rocks, when the time came, would be transferred in the precise order to honor the tradition. Our guide was watchful over all activities and governing the order of the plan. He named a gatekeeper for the lodge. The gatekeeper could not enter the lodge but would stand outside to let any other individual out. A line was forming outside the sweat lodge. After all this labor we were subdued and also a little frightened to go into this pitch black and very hot teepee. The female owner of the land stood next to the entrance of a medicine wheel, which was perhaps fifty feet in diameter. We were asked to walk around it three times and to listen for any possible messages.

The male owner of the land held a large shell containing some sweet smelling smoking herbs. He also had a large eagle feather and was waving it over the smoke and then over each one of us. This was called smudging and it was to cleanse and purify us before we entered the sacred space of the sweat lodge.

Our guide instructed us as to how we would enter the door and where to go and what to do once inside. There was very little room, no light at all, a red-hot pit with glowing rocks in the center, and we had to file in and find a place to sit. We were pressed together, side by side. The Chief entered last and closed the gate behind him. The "sweat" was divided into four stages of twenty minutes each. The gatekeeper was also the timekeeper. We were asked to silently form an intention or wish. We were informed that the power generated within these walls had far reaching influence and as long as our wish was from the heart, we could ask for anything. I do not remember what my wish was but I do know that I fervently wanted it. I had an intention to get it.

The Chief then began to chant a very low, mystical and ancient sound. The chant was not in English, so we could not follow along. As he chanted we began to imagine all sorts of visions playing around inside the lodge. Some of us began to cry, others giggled, others wanted to get out and did, and others went into deep meditation. I was one of the latter. At the twenty-minute break, the gatekeeper opened the door and everyone filed out, except me. Part of my consciousness knew what was happening but my intention, my wish, dictated that I remain in the sweat lodge the entire time. So I stayed put. During the break the rocks were checked and any possible leaks for light, then the gate closed for the rest of the break. For the ones going outside it was a chance to get out of the heat. They were being hosed off, given something to drink and some were running to the edge of the woods and throwing up.

I did not notice when the break was over, the gate was opened and the occupants filed in. I did not notice the next break, the next one or the last one. My meditation was deep and profound. I know that part of my intention was to gain understanding and increase my awareness of the Native American lore. I was serene to my core. The sweat was over and we lay down on the cool, lush, green grass. Some were singing the melody of the chant and others fell asleep. The ones who left after the first break were with the female owner of the land, preparing our feast. We had been there the entire day. We were all silent or speaking in low tones. We were not informed ahead of time to bring an offering to the Chief, but we found ourselves digging into our purses and pockets to reward him for his efforts. We later learned that an offer of tobacco or blue corn meal is offered to the land after a sweat, and also to the Chief. He was a most kind man, and we were such novices. Some were gathering their gear for the long drive home. The landowners offered the land as a place to sleep, right under the stars. Some did. I thought I had to get back home. I made it to the first motel a few miles down the highway.

I attended many sweats after that, some with the same Chief and landowners and some with other Chiefs in other parts of the country. Once, I was invited as the only white person and the only female, to attend a Native American healing ceremony. I was very honored and traveled a great distance to participate.

Upon arrival, I was greeted by the wives of the Indians and invited to the rear of the property where a fire and a circle were already in place. There was a Chief with the traditional headdress and other Chiefs with traditional, but smaller headdresses. I was briefly welcomed, barely acknowledged actually, and shown where to sit. The others had an animal skin upon which to sit, but I had none, so sat directly on the ground. We were in a tight circle.

The Chief lit some obviously homemade cigarettes and we all took one puff and passed it to the next person. After that, the Chief lit a pipe in a very ceremonial manner and passed it around. I do not know what was in that tobacco, but I felt fairly woozy afterwards.

I sensed a bit of tension in the circle. Everyone was quiet. I gathered it had something to do with me, the only female, and the only non-Indian. Actually, my great-great grandmother was full-blooded Cherokee, but it did not seem the time or place to mention that. The Chief looked at me and asked, "What did you see?" I definitely had experienced some visions, so I assumed that was what he meant. I started to speak. My voice sounded like someone else's. I raised both my arms up into the air and turned toward the Chief. I told him that I saw a great eagle come up through his body and out of his head. I went on and described this eagle spreading its wings to encompass our group and how the wings rapidly and loudly fluttered, as if to gift us with a message. The Chief again asked me, "What did you see?" I said that at the opposite end of the circle, but facing him, was the head of a wolf. The size of the head was as big as our circle and the mouth of the wolf was wide open. I told him that I seemed to be drawn into the wolf's mouth and the tongue was very red. I told him that I realized that the tongue was red because it was dripping with blood, the blood of his people. He asked no more, and he asked no one else to speak.

The Chief turned to another Chief beside him and motioned for him to hand me some things. This Chief got up and in sort of a crawl, came over to me. He was giving me two items. One was a pair of turquoise, beaded moccasins, with the insignia of the tribe on the toe. The other was a bag of fresh cedar leaves. He backed up and sat back down. The primary Chief looked around the group as if to let them know he was about to speak, with their agreement, and then began to speak to me again. He told me that the moccasins had been made for me because they understood that in my heart I walked the path of the Native American. The bag of fresh cedar leaves was from the sacred burial grounds of their people. I later recalled that I had visited that site when I was seven years old. The Chief went on to say that I was invited to be a Pipe Carrier. I knew what that meant. It was a very high, if not one of the highest honors to be bestowed. He told me where to get the material for the pipe and I was to carve it and to decorate it myself. I was overwhelmed and humbly grateful.

There were many other Native American experiences. At the time, I was also traveling to the Orient and studying ancient Tibetan, Chinese and Japanese holistic healing arts. I had also begun to go to India and to accept a Guru as my primary Teacher. I never did follow through and become a Pipe Carrier. To be asked was honor enough. I felt that even though I would continue to respect the Native American ways, I could not live it as they did. I am grateful for the experience and hold the Native Americans as high and sacred beings.

A Ho Mitaquissin
Blessings on all my relations.

Medicine Wheel

NORTH	Dec 22-Jan 19	Earth Renewal	Snow Goose	Birch Tree
	Jan 20-Feb 18	Rest & Cleansing	Otter	Quaking Aspen
	Feb 19-Mar 20	Big Winds	Cougar	Plantain
EAST	Mar 21-Apr 19	Budding Trees	Red Hawk	Dandelion
	Apr 20-May 20	Frogs Return	Beaver	Blue Camas
	May 21-Jun 20	Cornplanting	Deer	Yarrow
SOUTH	Jun 21-Jul 22	Strong Sun	Flicker	Wild Rose
	Jul 23-Aug 22	Ripe Berries	Sturgeon	Raspberry
	Aug 23-Sep 22	Harvest	Brown Bear	Violet
WEST	Sep 23-Oct 23	Ducks Fly	Raven	Mullein
	Oct 24-Nov 21	Freeze Up	Snake	Thistle
	Nov 22-Dec 21	Long Snows	Elk	Black Spruce

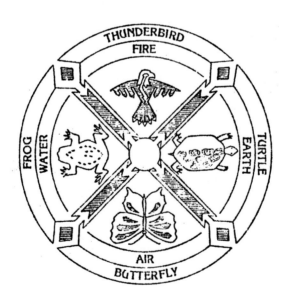

Reference Chart

Dec 22-Jan 19	Earth Renewal	Snow Goose	Birch Tree	
Jan 20-Feb 18	Rest & Cleansing	Otter	Quaking Aspen	
Feb 19-Mar 20	Big Winds	Cougar	Plantain	
Mar 21-Apr 19	Budding Trees	Red Hawk	Dandelion	
Apr 20-May 20	Frogs Return	Beaver	Blue Camas	
May 21-Jun 20	Cornplanting	Deer	Yarrow	
Jun 21-Jul 22	Strong Sun	Flicker	Wild Rose	
Jul 23-Aug 22	Ripe Berries	Sturgeon	Raspberry	
Aug 23-Sep 22	Harvest	Brown Bear	Violet	
Sep 23-Oct 23	Ducks Fly	Raven	Mullein	
Oct 24-Nov 21	Freeze Up	Snake	Thistle	
Nov 22-Dec 21	Long Snows	Elk	Black Spruce	

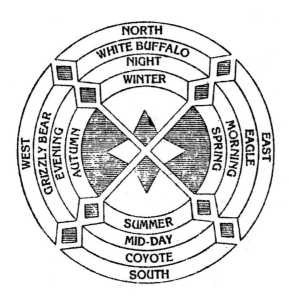

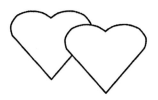

PROTECTION

Many individuals travel far and wide and consult with monks, ministers, psychologists, psychics, astrologers, seers of various types and talents, to discover why they were born. They want to know just what is the reason for being here? They are curious from their core as to what they are supposed to be doing on this planet and what their "path" is.

This has a simple answer: To serve God.

There are not too many folks who do not acknowledge some form of supreme being, higher power or creator of the universe. We were created by God to serve God, and in serving God we serve mankind. How can that be done? What is a clue? Where is a key to unlock this mystery for each individual? This also has a simple answer. Do what is directly in front of you. On some level, in some way, you planned your life. I am sure you have heard, probably from a chastising mother, that the angels up in the sky have everything about you written down. So it is. It is written. You have made your choices for your life. And, there is free will, so you may continue to make your choices. Oh, I know, you do not want to be responsible, you want someone to take care of you, make decisions for you, so you will not be to blame when something goes out of kilter. Sorry. It does not work that way. Someday, somehow, someway, you will have the realization that you are powerful, capable and have the privilege and the duty to serve mankind. Those who have this realization have even more responsibility because they must serve those who also have the realization, as well as those who have yet to come into this consciousness.

You may have negative experiences such as an eerie feeling while walking by a dark alley in a big city, being awakened in terror by a nightmare or someone actually threatening your peace of mind or your physical body. In order to serve God and mankind we must be in control of our faculties, our person and our surroundings. We must know of methods in which to protect ourselves, our family and our abode, whether permanent or temporary. Again, we have a duty to protect and we have the privilege to protect. Some will never know why it is our responsibility to make this world as protected as possible. This will raise the vibrations of the universe and make the world a better place in which to live.

There are as many protection modalities and methodologies as there are cultures and creeds. We may not label them as protection methods but we do employ ways and means that protect us and prevent negative energies from entering our space. Unschooled individuals may be feeling depressed and suddenly begin to sing or share an amusing story with a friend. The sound of music and laughter will raise the vibrations and negative energy will flee. Negative energies like us to be depressed or angry or just generally out of sorts. This creates weak areas in our energy system and the negativity is always searching for a place to nest. Then the depression, anger, anxiety, and more, get out of hand and become our way of life. In my stress management course, I encourage a discipline of positive thinking affirmations, grinning exercises that raise the endorphin level, breathing techniques for relaxation and the like.

The curious thing is that we often do not realize this is something that must be established as a daily discipline. Most of us are raised with some sort of punishment to make us behave. The other side of that is to reinforce positive behaviors with praise and gratitude. It takes structure and consciousness to move past any parental influences. Some folks think that laughing is rude, that singing, unless in a church choir, may be evil, and affirmations are of the new age ilk and to be avoided at all costs. Luckily research and studies are increasing awareness and providing understanding so that, hopefully, the world is moving into a higher consciousness.

Following will be an array of protection methods from different cultures and belief systems. Many I use in my healing procedures and some I have studied to increase my awareness and gain understanding. Always, always, always use a protection method for yourself before you begin a process for someone or something else. The first one is a combination protection process, designed by my daughter, Mandy, and taken from my *Reiki Touch* book, first published in 1988.

We were created by God in order to serve God by serving His children, mankind. Our reason and purpose for being on this planet is to serve one another.

A way we can do that is to protect our own energy so we can use it to help others and ourselves. How many times, either in a crowd or after a conversation with someone, have you felt drained and tired? If our energy is not contained or protected, we are basically putting our mental, emotional and physical energy on a silver platter and serving it as hors d'oeuvres.

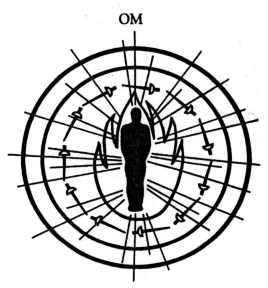

OM

I am the UNIVERSE	I am
I am the SPHERE	I am
I am the LIGHT	I am
I am the FLAME	I am
I am the SWORD	I am
I am the REFLECTION	I am
I am the UNIVERSE	I am

Observe the protection design. In the center you will see a human form. This is you, a family member or a consenting friend. Yes, permission is important before doing something for someone. If they are incapacitated in some way say a silent prayer to their heart and ask if you can do this for them. If it is property, ask the property. Everything has a consciousness and the property also has a heart.

- See that the human form is surrounded by various spheres or balls. At the top is the word, "Om," the primordial sound of the universe from which all other sounds derived. The word Om correlates with the first verse, "I am the Universe, I am." The words, "I am" are the words that connect and are the same as the word, Om. When this is spoken you are claiming your birthright, your existence, your place and your space on this planet. You are part of the whole, and the whole must have all of its parts. You are an integral part.

- The next line is "I am the Sphere, I am." Look at the second from the outermost sphere. This one is your own design. In what would you feel protected? Would you feel protected within a sphere of gold, rainbows, silver? Create your own sphere.

- The verse, "I am the Light, I am" acknowledges that you are light, love and energy. Claim it by stating it.

- "I am the Flame, I am" acknowledges the God of Fire, Agni, the Violet Flame of St. Germain and other holy fires and flames. This flame transmutes negative energy to positive energy by burning up anything that would prevent you from serving God and mankind.

- The ring of swords invokes St. Michael, the magnificent archangel of protection. We are all spiritual guardians. "I am the Sword, I am."

- "I am the Reflection, I am" can acknowledge the rays of light shining from your essence or you may create a visual image of a mirror reflecting out on the outermost sphere.

Close with gratitude, repeating, "I am the Universe, I am." Have confidence that you are now protected. Do this every morning (for the day) and every evening (for the night) for the rest of your life. Repeat it whenever you feel the need. Use it for your children or spouse, the workplace, an airplane for safe travel, for any reason you feel it is needed.

House and Land Clearing and Blessing

M any priests, Indian Chiefs, Brahmins, shamans, Kahunas and others are called upon to clear energies in a house, the land, and of course, people. I do not know of the complete and formal methodologies of the afore-mentioned, but I will share those that I have participated in and have used.

If a house is going to be cleared, a blessing should follow in order to ensure the clearing is transmuted from negative to positive energies. Many times you will read that a method is used three times. Why is that? For the body, mind and spirit; for the earth, water and sky, for many triplicate areas.

Depending on the size of the house and the scope of the land, have enough salt to surround the property. For a city residence I usually get two or three five pound bags of regular salt. I will position the bags at various distances so I will not have to retrace or depart my path. I tell the salt what I am using it for and thank it for assisting me in this process. Everything has a consciousness and gratitude brings you everything. Beginning at the north side of the property, I walk clockwise around the edge of the land and pour salt in an unbroken line all the way around the land three times.

For the house, I have previously placed a dish of fresh sage on windowsills for twenty-four hours. You can get this at health food stores. After that I take a coconut and beginning at the front or main entrance of the house, I offer the coconut to God and to all the directions. I blow on it three times. I tell the coconut what its mission is and offer gratitude for its work. Now I walk clockwise around the house, touching the coconut to each and every corner of the house saying "thank you." I walk around the house three times in this manner. The coconut is pulling negative energies out of the house. We now go inside the home, entering the front or main door. Again, clockwise, we walk through the house and touch the coconut to each doorway of each room. If I sense the necessity, I will go inside each room and circle it three times. I walk through the entire house a total of three times, all the time thanking the coconut for its mission. I depart the home through the same door in which I entered.

I have a plastic bag handy, large enough to completely hold the coconut. Usually there is a sidewalk, if not have a large rock ready at the outside entrance of the house. The coconut has absorbed negative energy outside and inside the house. You now raise the coconut high in the air, all the while offering gratitude, and bring the coconut down and smash it onto the sidewalk or rock. Collect all the pieces, large and small, and put them into the plastic bag. Also get all the dishes of sage and empty these into the same plastic bag. Close the plastic bag completely so nothing falls out. Within twenty-four hours take the plastic bag to a body of moving or running water, such as a river or an ocean, not a lake or pond. Empty the contents out of the bag and into the water, again offering gratitude. Burn the plastic bag.

After a day or night has passed, but within twenty-four hours, reenter the house. Put a special rice—jasmine, basmati, or rice with a blessed oil—in dishes on every windowsill. Pour the rice into the dishes while you are at that individual window. Pour generously so the rice generously overflows the dish. Ask the window to invite all good things into your home. Write your wish on a small piece of paper and place it under the dish. This could be health, happiness, prosperity, contentment, peace or whatever you desire. Remember to thank the rice and the window for its work. Gratitude brings you everything.

Maps

For a very large area of land, whether it has buildings on it or not, you use a map of the property. Sometimes it is a difficult terrain, has a creek or brook or underbrush, and an unbroken stream of salt is impossible. Cut out the perimeters or boundaries of the land so it is clear exactly what area is being addressed. Place the map on a flat surface in a room that will have no wind or direct sun or moonlight. Offer the work to the heavens, the earth and all the directions. Blow your divine prana onto the map three times. Ask a holy being to be with you and to guide and bless your work.

Begin at due north. You do have a compass, yes? Hold a bag of salt and let an unbroken line of salt surround the map three times. Say a prayer of some sort as you pour the salt. You may repeat "God is love" or an ancient, sacred Mantra, something in which you have total faith.

Put any kind of flower petals outside the ring of salt. Light a candle that will be guaranteed to burn for twenty-four hours. Offer gratitude to the salt, the flowers, the candle, and last but not least, the high being of your choice. Make sure that the windows are closed and covered and all air conditioning vents are directed away from the map. Now, leave it. Return to the room the next morning or evening after the twenty-four hours are over. Offer gratitude as you walk toward the map. Do not touch the map, the flower petals or the salt. Put your hands behind your back so you will not be tempted. Negative energies are great tempters.

Observe the map, the ring of salt and the flower petals. Amazingly, you will note that in some areas the ring of salt has been broken. The same may be true of the flower petals. The salt can also be wet and sometimes have a glue-like consistency. Since the room was sealed off and protected there is no natural or practical reason for this. Some energetic force has altered the integrity of the ring. Now, with a pen and paper, take notes as to the exact location where the salt and/or flower petal ring is disturbed.

Take a large bag of salt and flower petals out to the literal area of the property and pour the salt and scatter the flower petals, offering gratitude during the process. Return to the map and reinforce the broken areas with fresh salt and fresh flower petals. You will return the next day to again observe where, if any, areas of the salt perimeter or the flower petal ring are broken. If so, repeat the process. Do this for three days.

In Texas, as well as other states and countries, the cattlemen cherish their cattle. The ranches are sometimes hundreds and even thousands of acres in size. The monitoring of all the cattle is impossible and cattle rustling, or stealing, is common. One rancher hired me to protect his land and his cattle. Using this exact same process, his land was cleared and protected and the cattle rustling ceased.

General Supplies

Always have holy water prepared, to sprinkle on you, others, pets, the house, land. Just a sprinkle. Have an intention to protect and speak it out loud or silently. Yes, you were created in the image of God. You can do this. Your breath is divine. Some call the breath prana. Use a clean, clear glass and fill it with pure water. Clearing rituals are just that, rituals. So follow the instructions to the letter as much as is humanly possible. So, if I say a clean glass, I do not mean one in which you have just had a sip of tea or juice. Sterile. If I say a clear glass, use one that does not have decorations on it, anywhere. Pure water is bottled water, if possible. Organic is okay, distilled is better. Offer the water to the heavens, to the earth and to all the directions. Say out loud, "I offer this water to the heavens" and so on. Then, blow your own breath onto the water three times. Call upon a high and holy being such as God, Jesus, Mother Mary, your Guru, or whomever you deem holy. Ask this holy being to be with you as you do the entire process.

Even as these modalities and methodologies are being presented, realize that we are always protecting ourselves in one way or another. It is just common sense to move from discomfort to comfort. As knowledge and practice increases we will be more protected, have more obstacles removed and can do our chosen work with greater ease.

THE HO'OPONOPONO
Cleansing and Problem Solving

Following are some Huna processes done by the Kahuna teachers and healers in Hawaii. I had the great honor to study with Morna Simeona, an internationally known Kahuna. Morna was hired by governments to heal the land when it had been gouged by greedy miners or explorers. She knew how to communicate with the land, trees, water and everything created by God and to bring that into a state of harmony.

Always include the Lady of Freedom, the Unihipili of the United States of America, in your Ho'oponopono process. We include all Unihipilis of nations throughout the world and the universes.

- Divine Creator, Father, Mother, Child as one; I/We _____ my/our family, families, relatives and ancestors wish to do a HO'OPONO-PONO with _____.
- All my/our fears, errors, resentments, guilts, anger, violence, attachments with people, especially _____; places _____; past lives, home ties _____; that contribute to the cause of my/our problems.

Cleanse, purify, sever, cut and release all the negative and unwanted memories, blocks and energies we have created, accumulated and accepted from the beginning of our creation to the present and any others which relate or attach to this problem. Transmute all these unwanted energies to pure light.

We release them to pure light as they release us. We are set free!

And, it is done!

The Unihipili

The Unihipili, or the child within, reacts as an undisciplined, uncared, unloved aspect of us. It is also referred to as the serpent part of us.

The Unihipili or child can manifest itself as a lofty, refined part of our being or it can react as a destructive "serpent." The damage is multiplied and accentuated by "collective thought forms" of negative forces, ideas of criminals, thieves, prostitutes, politicians, money changers, slave drivers, hunger mongers, killers, murderers, abusers and the like.

The Unihipili may be referred to as a beloved child, young sister or brother, son or daughter which is a better type of relationship than any outside of one's framework. The Unihipili or child within us will respond or react according to our choices.

- CARE
1. Gently stroke the Unihipili from the top of the head down, with love, care and concern.
2. Hug the child gently, not a "bear hug." Bear hugs frighten the child.
3. Grasp the hand sweetly and gently stroke it.
4. Hold the shoulders and give unlimited love to the child.
5. Do extra breathing for the Unihipili before this process (breathing process explained at end of Unihipili).

Only with reverence will you be able to win your Unihipili's cooperation. When the Unihipili consents for you to continue, it will respond and you will be aware of this. Remember that your focus and attitude are being observed by him/her moment by moment.

1. Cleanse the self on behalf of the child or Unihipili. Heal the pains, scars and wounds gathered from everywhere in the ocean, land, air, animal kingdom, vegetable kingdom and all mankind from the beginning of creation to the present time and into the future.
2. The child is given a "jump suit" covering from head to toe. This is constructed of a soft, warm, blue cloth. The shoes and gloves are indigo in color. There is an abdominal, stretchable band seven inches wide with three hooks and eyes on the left side. This assures the child that the band is held firm and will not come undone. This has a three-fold purpose: Satisfaction, Security and Assurance.
3. Surround the child with indigo lined with ice blue. Ice blue has a touch of soft pink to give it compassion and love.
4. Communicate with the child to assure your constant, unending and unbroken love and support for all time. Wait until you sense that your child has received and accepted this. Be of good heart during the process.
5. Give your child or Unihipili a name, either KE-OLA, meaning life, or KA'LA, meaning Sun. Use a pendulum to get your child's preference and acceptance.

6. Offer gratitude to your child or Unihipili for the work together and consider it done.

UNIHIPILI BREATHING PROCESS: Have your intention in mind. Declare your breath as holy and powerful. Slowly inhale and exhale twenty-one times. This is for you. Now, focus on the object of your intention, in this case your child or Unihipili. Again, inhale and exhale twenty-one times. This will awaken and connect your child or Unihipili to you and the process will have the proper prana flow.

The Pillar of Peace of I

The Pillar of Peace of I is the ultimate result of balance within the individual's entire being. It is the radiance of the divine, the "I" within, attracting like vibrations.

When faced by or confronted with a person, place or thing that is threatening, negative or imbalanced then mentally imbue yourself in the Pillar of Peace of I and direct the Pillar of Peace of I to the individual, place or object from which the negativity or danger is located. The gross vibrations will melt and the emergence of peace or balance will occur. This is a mental projection only. The result is always positive.

When visiting, interviewing or traveling to and from various people, places and situations, cover yourself and the subject involved with the Pillar of Peace of I. The Pillar of Peace of I allows the expression of freedom and sets the subject free from vices, negativity, restrictions, limitations and prejudices. Above all, it brings balance where there was a separation of the subject from its own divinity that resides within.

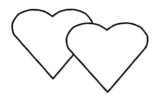

PSYCHOMETRY

Psychometry is a practice in which one explores the essence or spirit of a person, place or thing. This shamanic tool is employed to assist various agencies to locate a missing person or object. Many police and government offices will, in a nonpublicized way, utilize this talent to augment their work. I cannot, so far, claim to have miraculously found a lost child or someone's long, lost love. But I have found puppy dogs and jewelry and, even though perhaps considered small, it was important at the time to the owners.

A neighbor knocked on my door, distraught that her prize Pekinese puppy had wandered off. She was positive that the leash fit properly and that she had secured his play area. However, he was missing. She did not know that I had some talent in this area. After listening to her, and knowing this puppy personally, I asked her to take me to his play area. She thought that I was discounting her thoroughness in security and protection. This was not the case. I wanted an opportunity to psychically and supernaturally enter the puppy's vibrations or spirit body in order to communicate with him, and hopefully find him. I remained as casual as possible and asked normal type questions as to how old he was, his full name, the last time she saw him, the last time he was bathed, had a meal and questions of that type. All the questions bring me closer and further into his vibrations.

We entered his play area. I looked around for something I could hold to make a physical connection. There was a blanket upon which he slept. That was a good one. There were his feeding dishes too. These things would provide good vibrations. I suggested that we pray to God for the puppy's return. My neighbor was anything but spiritual and I also knew that she would have a skepticism that could prevent the vibrational leap to her puppy. However, she decided that prayer wouldn't hurt. I intentionally sat on his blanket and, without her noticing, held part of it in my hand. She nervously asked me if we had to pray out loud and if so, I had to do it. I reassured her that the prayers could be silent. She was relieved and so was I. I did count on God's help, no doubt, but I wanted to also specifically address the puppy.

As I held the pup's blanket I had a visual image, somewhat like a movie screen, in front of my third eye. I saw him very happily trotting along a side road that had a deep ditch with water in it. Taking deep breaths I followed him along this path. Two children on bicycles saw him and picked him up, put his tiny self into the bicycle basket and rode off to their home. The puppy was delighted. He was having a super adventure and lots and lots of attention. I smiled as I saw this moving image. The children took him inside and gave him some water. I saw a caring adult check him out. He was so cute and they all loved him.

I asked his vibrations to expand and to give me an image of the house where he was having such a good time. The house image was revealed. I moved closer to hopefully get any identifying numbers or address or street sign or something so the neighbor and I could find him.

I saw numbers, 4529 Willow Street. They were clear and, prayerfully, correct. After a few moments, instructing the puppy to stay where he was, and observing that his tired body went to sleep, I opened my eyes. The neighbor had earlier opened hers but was respectfully waiting for me. I took a deep breath and said that we had contacted God and I believed that prayers were answered, but that we could consider taking action and drive around the neighborhood to look for him. I offered to drive so I could be in control of the route.

We soon found the side road with the water-filled ditch. My neighbor began to cry and said that she knew he could not swim and what if he had fallen into the water. She wanted to stop the car at that moment and search the ditch. I knew he had passed the ditch so I gently suggested that we drive a bit more and then return to the ditch in a few moments.

I drove on looking for the Willow Street sign. I had to concentrate to remember the fuzzy numbers of the house.

At the end of the ditch the street that turned off it was named Willow. I thanked God and breathed a sigh of relief, along with a prayer to continue this good fortune. The little puppy had awakened from its nap. The mother wanted to instantly go out and place "Lost Puppy" signs around the neighborhood, but the children were enjoying him so much she delayed it for a while. The children took him out to the front yard and were having him fetch a small ball. There was much laughter and yapping.

I don't recall who reacted first, me or my neighbor. I think I saw him and I think she heard him. All in all, it did not matter. He was found. The mother and the children quickly realized the bond between the owner and pet and were happy he was back with his rightful owner. I was pleased too.

You can do this. It is not a magic trick. It is ownership of the energies that anyone can master. Merely claim it. Even though you cannot see the wind, you know it exists. Even though you cannot touch the sun, you can experience its warmth. There are invisible realities and you can bring them into conscious form. If something is lost, acquire something that has been close to that person, place or thing. Hold it and allow your vision to expand. Ask many questions, as that opens the energetic field and provides answers. When you are moving and searching you can call the lost object to you. You can call it as if you were calling a kitty. Literally say, "Here car keys, here car keys, here car keys."

You may also demand that the object just appear before you. Sometimes that can occur quickly and easily. Belief in the process is important. And last, but mandatory, thank the object for returning to you. Tell the object how important, perhaps even vital, it is to your life and implore it to stay with you. The expression and emotion of love energy is the main element to success in this endeavor.

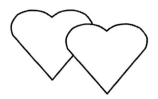

PSYCHIC SURGERY
Julia

Many years ago I had some lower back complications resulting from an injury. After braces and rehabilitation the doctors were considering exploratory surgery. This meant a scar the length of my spine. I was in the process of making a decision about this when my phone rang. A friend called to say there were some psychic surgeons in town and a film was to be shown that evening. It took several repeated efforts on her part to convince me to attend this event, but I ended up going.

The room was packed with normal, ordinary people. One was a neurosurgeon who had had his leg lengthened, another person who had experienced a successful tumor removal and other, to me, miracles. I listened to the testimonies and to the little, brown Filipino psychic surgeon and watched the film. What I saw on the screen was this intensely focused psychic surgeon aiming his quick fingers over an area of a patient's body and deftly entering the body, removing the diseased or imbalanced portion, then placing his full palms over his "incision," which closed the cut. All this was accomplished in less than a minute. It was like being at the circus watching a magician. I tried very hard not to be impressed.

After this presentation his assistant held up a registration form inviting anyone to go to Mexico for psychic surgery performed by Romy, the Filipino psychic surgeon. I was astonished at the hands swiftly moving through the air. The audience was filled with intense hope, desire and anticipation. Suddenly my hand lifted; it was as if someone tied a string to it, and like a puppet, I responded. My friend had promised me that it was cheaper than the traditional surgery, would leave no scars and no recuperation period. Too good to be true? I was going to find out.

A week later, instead of being in an ordinary operating room, I was in Mexico, about to experience psychic surgery. As I entered the room the surgeon and I made eye contact and smiled. It seemed that it was a smile I had known from lifetimes ago. The surgeon gave a spiritual type lecture impressing upon the patients that they had to believe in this or the disease would return. He was performing an extraction, but they had the responsibility of gaining understanding about why the disease happened in the first place. Only then would the body remain healed. No one paid any attention to that part. It was a spectacular moment, a phenomenon, and we were center stage. The psychic surgeon's instruments were his hands. In addition to that he had a peculiar smelling oil, little red plastic bowls, some cotton balls and a few ordinary disposable kitchen towels. I was lying on the treatment table and he passed an ordinary white sheet of typing paper over my body. This was his x-ray. To my skeptical amazement he began diagnosing all the items my doctor had described.

His assistant then used this not-so-fragrant oil and began massaging my back. The oil made my skin heat up and I later found that a diseased portion of a body had a higher heat and would, with this oil, rise to just under the surface of the skin. As this occurred, within a minute or less, the psychic surgeon would position his surgical fingers, dive in and remove the obstacles from my lower back. According to him this was some scar tissue and calcified bone. He put that into the little red plastic dish and someone flushed it down the toilet. He put his small, flat hand down over the incision, which closed it, and stepped back.

The assistant used the nonsterile cotton pads and kitchen towel to wipe off the blood and body fluids, finishing with the oil and a very brief massage. This all took about two or three minutes at the most.

Now, I could go take a walk on the beach or have lunch. He said not to do anything strenuous, such as water skiing, for two hours.

In the book, *Healers and the Healing Process,* by George Meeks, a chapter by William A. Tiller, PhD, formerly of Stanford University, explains that the ability to perform psychic surgery is a positive space-time and negative space-time, which stands for the physical and the etheric. This equation, using structure, chemistry, function, energies with mind, spirit and the divine, allows the extended surgery of the psychic surgeon to separate the cells and enter into the body. He further explained that it was this same reverse type principle that Jesus used to walk on water.

This psychic surgeon was seeing fifty-five patients twice a day; one hundred and ten each day, beginning at eight in the morning and finishing at six in the evening. He worked nonstop, as did his brother and the assistants. He would eat an enormous meal of fish and rice, which I later learned was his same meal three times a day, wherever in the world he was.

While there, I remembered that I had begun the "age forty astigmatism" and asked him if he could keep me out of eye glasses. He motioned for me to get onto the table again, and after a few seconds, completely removed my left eyeball from its socket. He spit on it, held it to his third eye, washed it off in Mexican tap water and put it back. He put his very warm and healing hand over the right eyelid and prayed. Years later my eyes are fine.

As I was lying there, wondering about the tap water, a little voice inside me said, "you can do this." I then heard my voice asking him if I could assist him. He said I had to read the seventeenth chapter of St. John in the New Testament. He said it was the most metaphysical chapter in the Bible. I had to stand, in front of everyone, with my newly healed eyes, and read this, three times, out loud. He then brought me over to a patient who had an imbalance just under her lower rib cage area. He showed me how to do the magnetic massage process. While I was massaging the area I felt a stringy or ropelike substance just under the skin. I motioned to Romy and told him what I felt. He said that if I could feel it I could go get it. I was confused, scared and unbelieving and protested that I could not "go get it."

He took my right hand, told me to point my forefinger at the body, and amazingly the skin opened. He instructed me to hold the skin open with my left hand and to remove, very slowly, the stringy, ripply substance with my right hand. After the material was removed he instructed me to slowly take my right hand out, now my left hand and to put my right hand flat, palm down, over the incision. I could sense the skin closing under my hand. It was as if it had never opened, yet there was blood and body fluid being wiped off by the assistant, and I had the same on my hands.

That was the first of many. Over a period of several years I traveled and worked with Romy and other psychic surgeons from the Philippines and from France. When I became tired he instructed me to stand in the sunlight. He said for me to ask the sun's light and warmth to enter and rejuvenate me. He said for me to turn around three times counterclockwise and then turn around three times clockwise. I use this method to this day.

During this time I began to study Reiki, a new healing technique. Psychic surgery was a magnetic healing form that would draw an imbalanced or diseased part of the body to the surface of the skin. Reiki was a form of energy healing which would address the source and acknowledge the innate perfection of the body. Reiki would support the cell memories in reinstating this perfection. This was a different and opposite modality. In my mind I had been wondering if I would devote my life to psychic surgery. It was illegal in the United States and I had grave concerns about that segment of it.

The focus and action of psychic surgery was counterproductive to the nonmagnetic force of Reiki. Psychic surgery removes the effect. Reiki removes the cause. The energies in my body were doing cartwheels. I became nauseated, had headaches and could not focus. I had to make a decision. I chose Reiki. I am grateful to Romy and to the other psychic surgeons with whom I trained and served. I am grateful perhaps in some way, to have been a part of instilling hope and understanding in the patients who chose and still choose psychic surgery.

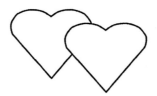

REIKI TOUCH™ THERAPY
Julia

This chapter begins with expressing my gratitude to my Guru, to all the ascended Tibetan masters, to Dr. Usui, Dr. Hayashi and Mrs. Takata, the most recent ascended Reiki Masters. Included in this gratitude is the current Grand Master of Reiki, Phyllis Lei Furumoto. Next, the long and honored list of students of Reiki: the Reiki Masters, Reiki Professional Degrees, and the first and second levels of Reiki. They are all vital levels of attainment, each having its own degree of mastery. You may enjoy reading about this in detail in my book, *Reiki Touch.*

In the late seventies and early eighties, I was very interested in healing modalities and was very much drawn to the Far East to explore these techniques. One evening, as part of a holistic healing group, I walked into a room and observed something to which I had not yet been introduced. A fully dressed man was lying on a treatment table and a woman was gently resting her hands on this man's back. The man and the lady were communicating and sometimes were even lightheartedly joking. Her hands were not moving at all and the man seemed not to mind. This nonmovement, the lack of focus and concentration appeared very unprofessional and foreign to any healing technique I had known. In a judgmental voice I inquired as to what she was doing. Her answer was brief: Reiki. I did not ask her to explain what Reiki was, but insisted that it could not work due to the lack of focus and the obvious camaraderie. In addition to that, her hands were not moving.

She was silenced by my verbal disbelief but the man was not. He said that he had been experiencing some bad pain in his back and there was some heat and energy coming out of her hands. He said that even after a few minutes his back felt better. I was not at all convinced and also wanted to hear no more of it.

Soon after I returned to the states I observed a poster announcing a Reiki Master coming to my city to teach this "whatever it was." My ire was up. My intention when enrolling was to blow the cover and expose this so-called healing art as a hoax. I was quite adamant about this. You have heard the saying, "The bigger they are, the harder they fall"? I was being set up, big time.

The class held about a dozen or so curious people. My role was to gather information so this could be quelled, and quickly. The teacher was older, wise and astute. My attitude was soon revealed and an unexpected tact was presented to me. The teacher suggested that I be the assistant and aid in various tasks required to make the class flow more smoothly. Give a renegade a purpose and the renegade is no longer a renegade. My ego was given a boost, so the teacher must not be all bad.

Regardless of the teacher and my attitude, the energy of Reiki took me over. I was humbled, respectful and introduced into an ancient discipline, which totally fascinated me. It was sweet, gentle and noninvasive but was also very powerful and energetic. Two days after I finished that weekend seminar I printed up my business cards announcing that I was a Reiki practitioner. There was more to this, of course, but this was my first act of acceptance.

A medical doctor happened to be a member of this same class and he invited me to become part of his traditional medical team. He wanted to offer a wider range of healing modalities to his patients. I accepted his offer and for over two years had a practice there. During this time I furthered my studies and about three years later also became a Reiki Master. In this ancient, 3000-year-old lineage, vows are taken to make Reiki the prime focus for life.

For the next twenty years I traveled the globe many times, teaching and practicing this amazing holistic healing technique. I say amazing, because to this day, I am still a full-time Reiki Master, and I am constantly experiencing amazing results from this simple, anyone can do it, Reiki.

Soon, great interest was generated in the traditional medical communities regarding holistic medicine. Indeed, every hospital in the nation was mandated to have a minimum of one office or one practitioner of holistic medicine. There were many invitations from universities for speaking engagements, seminar presentations and also research. Research was and is a fascinating blend of the holistic and the traditional medical field. Many wonderful positive results have been obtained and published revealing the successful marriage of eastern and western philosophies of wellness.

I travel less and write more now. Consultations fill my calendar. There are the new, the curious and the ones who are mandated to be exposed to holistic medicine. Reiki is noninvasive, requires no ingestion of anything at all, is similar to taking a nap on a comfy sofa, and anyone can do it, even small children. The bottom line is that it "works." Try it!

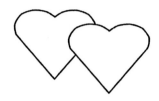

Orange Everywhere

Orange everywhere
Everywhere orange
All around
To the right, to the left
Up and down, back and forth
Orange everywhere
Everywhere orange

Orange everywhere
Everywhere orange
Beyond the orange is the gold
And, they are the same
The orange is the gold
The gold is the orange
Orange everywhere
Everywhere orange

Orange everywhere
Everywhere orange
Orange is love
Love is all

All is love and all is orange
Orange everywhere
Everywhere orange

Orange everywhere
Everywhere orange
Orange is light
Light is truth
Orange is light and truth
Orange everywhere
Everywhere orange

Orange everywhere
Everywhere orange
She is orange
She is gold
She is love
She is all
She is light
She is truth
Orange everywhere
Everywhere orange

Julia Carroll, 1994

BLESSING
Julia

Plato said, "Know Thyself."

This is a creed, a doctrine, a prayer and more; to be contemplated and acted upon. I invite you to spend your moments, awake and asleep, with evolutionary and enlightening thoughts, words and actions. Be true to yourself. In being true to yourself you will also be true to others. Endeavor to be responsible and accountable for all actions.

With humility, please accept my blessings.

On this day and forever more, for all eternity, may you have wonder-filled days and nights. May your dreams become realities. May the bright sun be reflected in your smile and the soft moon reflected in your mind. May each and every aspect of your body, mind and spirit be blessed. May the Gods and Goddesses of prosperity and abundance bestow grace upon you for your self-efforts. May the angels of mercy guard your health and your well-being. May you be protected from harm in all ways at all times and in all places.

May you enjoy empowerment, encouragement, peace and clarity of mind, astute and wise decisions, boldness, humility, intuition, love, understanding, sweetness, honor and self-approval. May all your wishes come true.

May you have a constant connection with your God. May you rest in the reassurance of being a child of God. May the effulgent joy of the heavens reverberate in your body, mind and spirit. Love your God, love yourself and love others with courage, steadfastness, self-effort and grace.

So be it.

AFTERWORD
Rosa Glenn Reilly

When I met Julia Carroll twenty years ago, neither of us immediately recognized that we walked similar paths. Julia was a blond with a warm Texas accent, brought up as a Baptist, and teaching Reiki Touch™ at my healing center. I was a Hispanic Catholic woman from Chile promoting alternative healing modalities. We discovered that we strongly believed in the innate power of an individual to heal themselves. This sometimes is with the assistance of an experienced practitioner. We also had similar concerns regarding the boundaries of allopathic medicine and the promise and personal empowerment of alternative approaches.

As recently as the eighties, yoga was considered radical, meditation was suspect, and healing through touch was considered a phenomena practiced under tents in rural backwoods. Certainly touch healing would not be found in Houston, Texas, a sophisticated urban city in the shadow of the world's largest medical center. However, this is exactly where we were, teaching an ever-growing population who never imagined themselves to be pioneers of the largest healthcare revolution of our time.

As a young child in Chile, I was exposed to a wide variety of folk healing practices. I was born two months premature, weighing only three pounds, slept in a shoebox and was fed breast milk with an eyedropper. Out of desperation to keep me alive, my grandmother became a self-taught healer. In addition, prayers, a warm and quiet environment and many loving hands were constant each day. My grandmother later traveled by boat, all over the world to explore alternative remedies. She later wrote a book on medical childcare that has been a mainstay in Chilean households for over forty years.

The indigenous Indian women, known as spiritualists, or curanderos, raised me. Even before the age of six I was taught to "place my hands here and ask God to help" or "take a few of those green herbs and sticks, boil them and drink them to get well." I was taught that it was a God-given gift and it was understood, as an exchange of energy, for the treated individual "to do something good in return."

Julia was the first person I met in the United States who regarded healing as a natural part of life. She held the same curiosity and determination as the women in my immediate and extended family. Julia had the fervor to teach and keep the integrity of the practices. She regards herself as a healer without believing herself special because of it. Julia is special because of who she is, and how she walks her path, which was presented to her at such a young age.

The ground she has broken in professional circles makes her unique because she opens doors for others to follow. Because of what Julia has done, this book will not be considered "fringe medicine." She is special because she believes that you are, and I am, and we all have unlimited capabilities we can access to use for ourselves and for others. This results in the betterment of those around us as we allow the opening of our eyes and hearts.

Julia has generously described her healing experiences over the past five decades. She has taken you, the reader, on a detailed journey of what she faces when someone enters her office for healing, sometimes as a last resort. You have witnessed her research and travels as she has learned from others. The greatest teacher is the greatest student. You will observe, as the wisdom in these pages permeate your being, a vast difference in your life.

Take a moment to connect with your inner stillness and listen to the innate wisdom. In what way do these pages speak to you? Should you follow the path of a healer? Do you now have information from which to heal your own body, mind and spirit? Can you support the complementary and alternative medical approaches to well being? Now, it is your turn to "do something good in return," as the curanderos would say. By reading this book you have been changed and healed in a way personal only to you. Take this energy and use it with great love.

Rosa Glenn Reilly
Founder, The Spectrum Center
Houston, Texas

JULIA CARROLL, BFA, MA, ATC

Fine Arts, Behavioral Sciences, Art Therapy, Reiki Touch™ Therapy

CURRICULUM VITAE

P.O. Box 270957 • Houston, Texas 77277 • Email: jcarroll@wt.net

EDUCATION

• 2001 University of Houston	MA Behavioral Science, Psychology
• 2001 University of Houston	Post-Graduate, Art Therapy Degree
• 1984 Houston Community College	Psychology courses
• 1963 Lousiana College	BFA, Fine Arts, Art
• 1959 McNeese State University, Louisiana	Liberal Arts courses

CURRENT POSITIONS

- Faculty: Psychology Department: University of Houston
- President and Founder: Reiki Touch Institute of Holistic Medicine™
- Professional Mediator: Cross-cultural Business; Family and Domestic

FORMER POSITIONS

- 1998-1999: Continued research projects (see research below)
- 1996-1998: Texas Children's Hospital, CIVITAS Child Trauma Program. Utilizing holistic medical treatments of Reiki Touch™ Therapy on severely maltreated children. Under the auspices of Bruce D. Perry, MD, PhD, Chief of Staff for Psychiatry and Neurology.
- 1974-1982: Owned and operated real estate agency; Houston, Texas.
- 1968-1974: Art educator in public and private schools; High School and Junior High.
- 1965-1968: Auburn University, Alabama; Art faculty in Fine Arts and Graphic Design.

RESEARCH

- 1999-2001: Department of Medicine, University of Arizona, Tucson, Arizona; Designed. and organized research study entitled "Efficacy of Reiki Touch™ Therapy in Reducing Pain, Nausea and Anxiety associated with Radiation and Chemotherapy Treatments for Patients with Cancer."

In association with Andrew Weil, MD, Integrative Medicine Program.

- 2000: University of Houston, in conjunction with Texas Children's Hospital, Houston, Texas; Study entitled "Art Therapy Modalities with Severely Maltreated Foster Children."
- 1998-1999: Kessler Rehabilitation Research Center, New Jersey; Consultant for Reiki Study entitled "Effect of Energy Healing on Post-Stroke Rehabilitation Patients."
- 1996-1998: University of Texas Health Science Center; Designed and managed study entitled "Reiki Touch™ Study on TMJ." (Temporomandibular dysfunctions)
- 1995-1996: University of Texas Health Science Center; Designed and managed study entitled "Triangulated Evaluation of Reiki Healing."
- 1994-1995: Harvard Medical School, Community Health Program; Designed and consulted study entitled "Reiki Touch™ Therapy with Psychiatric Patients with Severe Chronic Pain." Study was replicated three times.

CONFERENCE PRESENTATIONS

- 2000-2001: University of Houston, Houston, Texas; Presentation: "Student Views of Holistic Medicine Compared to Traditional Medicine."
- 1999-2000: Department of Medicine, University of Arizona, Tucson, Arizona, in conjunction with Andrew Weil, MD, Integrative Medicine Program. Seminars entitled "Reiki Touch™ Therapy as Related to Cancer Research."
- 1998-1999: Harvard Medical School Teaching Facility, Dana Farber Cancer Institute, Boston, Massachusetts; Seminars entitled "Reiki Touch™ Therapy as Related to Cancer Treatment."
- 1998-1999: Brigham and Women's Hospital, Boston, Massachusetts; Seminars entitled "Reiki Touch™ Therapy as Related to Cancer Treatment."
- 1997: University of Texas School of Nursing: Presentation, "Touch Therapies in Particular addressing Reiki Touch™ Therapy."
- 1996: University of Texas School of Nursing: Presentation, "Holistic Therapies including Reiki Touch™ Therapy."
- 1995: (Selected) Wives of Ambassadors of the United Nations, New York City, New York; Advanced Seminar, "Reiki Touch™ Therapy."
- 1995: Reiki Masters in Global Reiki Alliance: Curacao, Dutch West

Indies; Presentation, "Reiki Touch™ Therapy."
- 1995: Reiki Masters in Montreal, Canada; Presentation, "Reiki Touch™ Therapy.
- 1994: (Selected) Members of the Theatre and the Arts, London, England; Presentation, "Reiki Touch™ Therapy."
- 1994: Health Connections Company; Hong Kong; Presentation and Seminars, "Reiki Touch™ Therapy and Spirituality."
- 1989: Health and Spirituality Conference, Vancouver, British Columbia; Presentation, "Reiki Touch™ Therapy."
- 1986: Waidongong Wealth Conference, Taipei, Taiwan; Presentation, "Reiki Touch™ Therapy.
- 1986: American Imagery Association, Chicago, Illinois; Presentation, "The Dragon Within."
- 1986: University of Houston, Houston, Texas; Women's Annual Conference, Presentation, "Own Your Power."
- 1985: Unity World Conference, Houston, Texas; Presentation, "The Power of Inner Healing."
- Numerous other speaking engagements globally.

PUBLICATIONS

- Author of *Reiki Touch* book; First Edition: 1988. Second Edition: 1995. Third Edition in process. Distributed by New Leaf Distributing Company, Atlanta, Georgia.
- Author of numerous newspaper and magazine articles.
- Featured in major newspapers such as Hong Kong Standard Sunday Magazine, May 1, 1994; Mexico City's largest newspaper in 1992, 1993, and 1994. Houston Chronicle Lifestyle Section, September 20, 1987. Also smaller national papers.
- Acknowledged, cited and quoted (from her book, *Reiki Touch*), in medical journals as follows:
- 1992: Doctoral Dissertation for University of Texas School of Public Health: "Conceptual Models of Healing and Health: An Ethnography of Healers and Nurses," by Joan Engebretson, DrPH. Numerous articles written from this dissertation from which Julia Carroll is acknowledged, cited and quoted from her book, *Reiki Touch.*
- 1996: Qualitative Health Research, An International, Interdisciplinary Journal. Volume 6. No. 2.
- 1996: *IMAGE Journal of Nursing.* Volume 28, No. 2.

- 2001: Journal of Advanced Nursing, Blackwell Science Ltd., Volume 33, No. 4.
- 2002: Alternative Therapies, A Peer-Reviewed Journal, Volume 8, No. 2.
- 2002: *Emerging Lifestyles* Magazine, Volume 4, No. 12.

- Additional -

- 2001: Designed curriculum for university level art therapy course, taught by Julia Carroll, University of Houston, Houston, Texas.

- Memberships -

- AAUP American Association of University Professors
- AATA American Art Therapy Association (Certified Art Therapist)
- AASMI American Association for the Study of Imagery
- ABA Association for Behavioral Analysis
- WSA World Speakers Association^{SM}

"FRINGE MEDICINE"
CURRICULUM VITAE

- Old and New Testament Courses, Lousiana Baptist College; 1960-1963
- Prosperity Seminars, New York, San Francisco, Houston; 1975-current
- Omega Seminar, Leonard Orr: Houston, Texas; 1976
- Sound and Color, William David: Sedona, Arizona; 1978
- Meditation Seminar, William David: Sedona, Arizona; 1978
- Psychic Phenomena; Leonard Parsons: London, England; 1978-1980
- Mystery Schools (4), Jean Houston: Houston and Austin, Texas; 1980-1985
- Reiki I, II, Reiki Master; 1982-Current
- Psychic Surgery; Mexico, Orient, USA; 1982-1988
- Physio-Spiritual-Etheric-Body Healing, David Jarrell: Houston, Texas; 1983
- Master of Seven Rays, David Jarrell: Miami, Florida; 1983
- Trager Body Movement, Milton Trager, MD: Houston, Texas; 1983
- Dreams and Symbols, Carl Jung Center: Houston, Texas; 1983
- Native American Studies, Florida, Tennessee, Texas; 1983-1987
- Aquarian Old and New Testament Studies, Houston, Texas; 1984

- Divine Feminine Seminar, Mary Elizabeth Marlow: Virginia Beach, Virginia; 1984
- Aura Studies and Psychic Healing, Olivia Crawford: New Orleans, Louisiana; 1984
- Cancer Visualization Seminars, Carl Simonton, MD: Houston, Texas; 1984
- Emerging Woman Seminar, Mary Elizabeth Marlow: New Orleans, Louisiana; 1984
- IA, Integrative Awareness Seminar, Consuela Newton: Chicago, Illinois; 1984
- Pranic Healing, Earnestine Michenor: Baltimore, Maryland; 1984
- Chi Gong; John Song and Herbert Yuang: 1985-1986
- Shamanism, Hilary Karp, PhD: University of Houston; 1985
- Shamanistic Seminar, Chuck Lawrence: University of Houston; 1985
- Shaman Studies, Stanley Krippner, PhD: Houston, Texas ;1985
- Reincarnation, Psychic Development, Carol Parrish-Harra: Tahlequah, Oklahoma; 1985
- Exorcism Rites Studies, Barbara L. McCullough: Chicago, Illinois; 1985
- Meditation Courses, Gurumayi Chidvilasananda®: Globally; 1985-Current
- Huna Seminars (3), Morna Simeona with Serge King: Houston, Texas; 1985-1987
- Exorcism Rites Studies, Carol Parrish-Harra: Tahlequah, Oklahoma; 1986
- Wai Don Gong, Taiwan, Republic of China; 1986
- American Association for Study of Mental Imagery, Chicago, Illinois; 1986
- Master Mind Series, Jack Boland: Houston, Texas; 1986
- Psychic Protection, Sandee Mac: Houston, Texas; 1986
- Past Life Studies, Sandee Mac: Houston, Texas; 1986
- Astrological Numerology, David Jarrell: Coral Gables, Florida; 1986
- Twelve Powers of Man, Pat Pennington: Houston, Texas; 1986
- Tantra Seminar, Nellie Grose, MD: Houston, Texas; 1987
- Lazarius Seminar, Lazarius: Atlanta, Georgia; 1987
- Reiki Training for Dolphins, Dolphin Research Center: Florida Keys; 1987
- INTA, International New Thought Alliance, Presenter: Houston, Texas; 1987

- Return to the Heart Seminar, Bill Ferguson: Houston, Texas; 1988
- Crystal Uses Seminar, Randall Baer: Houston, Texas; 1988
- Authored *Reiki Touch* book, 1988-Current
- Creative Visualization Seminars, Shakti Gawain: Houston, Texas; 1988
- Breakthrough Seminar, Dr. John DeMartini: Houston, Texas; 1990
- Quantum Healing Seminar, Deepak Chopra, MD: Houston, Texas; 1990
- Collapsing and Coning Seminar, Dr. John DeMartini: Houston, Texas; 1990
- Feng Shui Studies for Home Balancing; Sandee Mac: Houston, Texas; 1994
- Feng Shui Studies for Financial Prosperity; Joani Nunez: Houston, Texas; 1999
- Integrative Medicine Principles, Andrew Weil, MD: Austin, Texas; 2000
- Holistic Behavioral Science, Joan Borysenko, PhD: Austin, Texas; 2000
- An Evening with Deepak, Deepak Chopra, MD: Austin, Texas; 2000
- Spirituality and Consciousness, Tulsi Saral, PhD: University of Houston in Texas; 2001
- Creativity, Irene E. Corbit, PhD: University of Houston in Texas; 2001
- Educational Art Therapy, Jerry Fryrear, PhD: University of Houston in Texas; 2001
- Aging, Howard Eisner, PhD: University of Houston in Texas; 2001
- Esoteric Christianity I & II, Carol Parrish-Harra, PhD: Tahlequah, Oklahoma; 2005

NOTES

Printed in the United States
36620LVS00001B/15-24

9 780615 129136